Get into
Pharmacy School
Rx for Success!

Third Edition

Other Kaplan Books for Pharmacy Students
Kaplan PCAT 2012–2013
Kaplan Medical NAPLEX

Get into Pharmacy School

Rx for Success!

Third Edition

William Douglas Figg, PharmD, MBA and Cindy H. Chau, PharmD, PhD

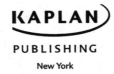

KAPLAN

PUBLISHING

New York

© 2011 by Cindy H. Chau and William D. Figg

Published by Kaplan Publishing, a division of Kaplan, Inc.
395 Hudson Street
New York, NY 10014

Printed in the United States of America

10 9 8 7 6 5 4 3 2 1

ISBN-13: 978-1-60714-833-3

Kaplan Publishing books are available at special quantity discounts to use for sales promotions, employee premiums, or educational purposes. For more information or to purchase books, please call the Simon & Schuster special sales department at 866-506-1949.

TABLE OF CONTENTS

Part Three: APPLYING TO PHARMACY SCHOOL—NAVIGATING THE APPLICATION PROCESS

Part Four: PREPARING FOR YOUR CAREER IN PHARMACY

Part Five: FINANCING YOUR DEGREE

Part SIX: RESOURCES

Authors

Dr. Cindy H. Chau received her BS degree from UCLA and PharmD and PhD degrees from the University of Southern California School of Pharmacy. She completed a post-doctoral fellowship at the NIH. Dr. Chau is a scientist within the National Cancer Institute.

Dr. William Douglas Figg, PharmD, MBA, received his BS in Pharmacy from Samford University and his doctoral degree from Auburn University. He also received an MBA degree from a combined program at Columbia University and the London Business School. He completed a post-doctoral fellowship at the University of North Carolina School of Pharmacy. Dr. Figg is a section head within National Cancer Institute.

Acknowledgments

We would like to acknowledge CAPT Pamela Schweitzer, PharmD, CAPT Gary W. Blair, DPh, MPA, PP, and CAPT Michael Clairmont for contributing to the section on pharmacy careers in the U.S. Public Health Service in chapter 16.

We would also like to express our grateful thanks to Sandy Ockers and Erika Smith for their assistance in compiling the pharmacy school statistics in the resource section.

How to Use This Book

This guidebook will help you prepare for pharmacy school by navigating you through the application process and providing you with unlimited resources you can utilize along the way. As a potential applicant, you need to first be familiar with pharmacy by knowing what the profession entails, how and where pharmacists practice, what programs are available at the different colleges and schools of pharmacy, and most importantly, whether this is the right field for you.

Once you have made the commitment to pursue a pharmacy career, you should plan ahead and determine the necessary steps you'll need for the application process. Applying to pharmacy school is like applying to any graduate (law or business school) or professional program (medical or dental school)—it requires careful planning and a significant amount of time and effort for this preparation.

This guidebook will introduce you to the profession, provide detailed guidance on how to apply to pharmacy school, give you a glimpse of what to expect while you're in school, and point you in the direction of the various pathways you can take as a pharmacist. In the last section of the book, you will find entering class statistics on different pharmacy programs across the nation, a timetable for applicants, and other resources that will help you adequately prepare and apply for pharmacy school.

We have designed this book for a range of audiences: the high school or college student interested in pursuing a pharmacy degree, the pharmacy student preparing for post-pharmacy school opportunities, the pharmacist exploring other avenues to pursue within the pharmacy profession, the guidance counselor looking for pharmacy school statistics, or any other individual seeking to learn more about the field of pharmacy.

PART ONE

Is Pharmacy School for You?

CHAPTER 1

Introduction to Pharmacy

Pharmacy is a dynamic profession that offers great flexibility and a challenging, yet rewarding career—pharmacists play an integral part of the health professional team. Today's pharmacists are also facing many great opportunities for expanded practice scopes, from community pharmacy to hospital pharmacy to academia and more. (We'll cover myriad options available to pharmacy school graduates in chapter 16.) This constant evolving and changing of roles has created the need for interdisciplinary training in areas beyond that of the traditional entry-level pharmacist.

WHAT IS PHARMACY?

Pharmacy (a word derived from the Greek word meaning "drug") is a licensed health profession charged with ensuring the safe use of medication. Traditionally, it is the art and science of preparing and dispensing drugs and medicine. However, more recently, pharmacy has transitioned to a field that encompasses not only medication distribution and use but also other services related to patient care including clinical practice, medication management, and drug information. To practice pharmacy in the United States, all new graduates need to hold a Doctor of Pharmacy (PharmD) degree and pass a state licensure examination. (See chapter 14 for more information on this exam.)

With the profession of pharmacy comes a good deal of respect. Because pharmacists are the most accessible healthcare providers and experts on medication management, they have consistently been ranked among the most trusted of professionals. When people enter their pharmacies for medicine, they usually leave with lots of information and advice. Pharmacists have the capacity to reach out to the community to provide knowledge about proper medication use, and when they do so, people are usually impressed when they get more than they ever expected from their pharmacists.

A PROFESSION ON THE RISE

It is a good time to be a pharmacist. According to data from the Bureau of Labor Statistics, the pharmacy profession continues to be on the rise based on salary and job prospects. The 10-year job growth rate, from 2006 to 2016, is projected to be at 22%, which is increasing much faster than the average for all occupations. The increasing demand for pharmacists is likely driven by the growing elderly population who typically have more complicated drug regimens and use more prescription drugs. As the use of prescription drugs increases, demand for pharmacists will grow in most practice settings; thus, excellent opportunities are expected for pharmacists over the 10-year projection period.

Pharmacist salaries are high and will likely rise even higher. According to the U.S. government's newly released Occupational Employment and Wage Estimates, based on 2009 data, the typical pharmacist makes an average of over six figures a year. Pharmacist salaries continue to climb despite the recent U.S. economic woes that caused millions of Americans to lose their jobs and pushed unemployment to levels unseen in decades.

Even with such positive aspects of the profession on the rise, the shortage of pharmacists continues to be an important issue for the healthcare industry. Current data suggests that there are not enough pharmacists to meet this existing demand. Faced with the rapidly growing consumer demand for prescription drugs, a sufficient supply of pharmacists is needed to ensure safe and accurate medication distribution. Pharmacists provide essential information on the safe use of drugs and help patients manage their diseases.

As such, the recruitment of students for the pharmacy profession remains a critical need. To meet this demand for competent, qualified pharmacists, more and more pharmacy schools have cropped up over the past few years. By 2011, more than 120 pharmacy schools are set to open across the United States that are recruiting students for enrollment in their programs. Even with this surge in the creation of new pharmacy schools, there will continue to be a shortage of pharmacists through 2030, with the estimated shortfall rising to 38,000 pharmacists, according to a report on the pharmacist workforce released in December 2008 by the Department of Health and Human Services.

THE CHANGING ROLE OF THE PHARMACIST

Pharmacists have become increasingly valuable to the healthcare system by contributing their expertise in the area of disease state management. Collaborative **medication therapy management** (MTM) approaches place the pharmacist at the forefront of healthcare delivery. (MTM is further discussed in chapter 2.) As healthcare continues to evolve, pharmacists' assessments (on drug therapy or drug allergies, for example) and responsibility for monitoring patients' drug use and therapy continue to improve patient care and might ultimately result in increased savings for the healthcare system. With aging baby boomers, an increase in the elderly population, and the implementation of Medicare Part D, more and more consultant pharmacists are called upon to provide MTM. As such, the growth and advancement of the profession will continue to flourish and change as the scope of pharmacists' practices continue to expand.

While pharmacists are traditionally reimbursed for the prescriptions they fill, they now can also be reimbursed for providing clinical services like MTM. Additionally, the new healthcare reform act, officially called the Patient Protection and Affordable Care Act, recognizes the importance of MTM with several grants and pilot programs to implement medication management services in the treatment of chronic diseases.

WHAT CAN A CAREER IN PHARMACY LEAD TO?

The opportunities in the profession of pharmacy are second to none.

Community Pharmacy

In many respects, community pharmacists represent the first line of healthcare. Practicing pharmacy in this setting involves dispensing medications, monitoring for side effects and interacting drugs, and providing important counseling services such as the proper selection of over-the-counter medications, herbal products, and/or referral to other healthcare providers when warranted. This is commonly seen as the practice of pharmacy at the retail store in your local community. Community pharmacies are divided into two types. The typical chain drugstore consists of pharmacies such as Walgreens, CVS, Rite-Aid, and the like. There are also independent community pharmacies that are pharmacist-owned and privately held.

The Pharmaceutical and Biotechnology Industry

This category represents any of the drug or biomedical companies and includes such companies as Amgen, AstraZeneca, Eli Lilly, Genentech, Johnson & Johnson, Merck, and Pfizer, for example. As a pharmacist, you can be involved in the sales & marketing of a Food and Drug Administration (FDA)-approved drug by working on marketing reports, or you can assist in developing packaging options and/or programs to help market the drug. You can participate in the research and development (R&D) of a new drug from basic discovery in a laboratory setting to using your knowledge on pharmacy and science in developing the delivery systems or formulation design of a new drug. It may also interest you to work in the Regulatory department handling the regulatory and legal requirements of the biomedical product development. Or, you may decide that you are better suited for the Clinical Development division where you will be involved with the day-to-day operations of monitoring the drug testing in clinical trials. Whatever area within the biomedical industry you are interested in, a degree in pharmacy will definitely prepare you for these various opportunities.

Academia

If you enjoy teaching, you can become one of the faculty members working in the nation's colleges and schools of pharmacy. You will not only be involved in teaching the next generation of pharmacy students, but also in conducting research in any area of pharmacy practice or science discipline for which you develop an interest.

Hospital Pharmacy

Pharmacists working in this environment are members of the hospital healthcare team and work directly with physicians, nurses, and patients. You will have various job responsibilities, including dispensing medications, providing drug information, performing drug dosing and monitoring, or compounding sterile products for patients such as total parenteral nutrition and other medications given intravenously.

Health Insurance Industry/Pharmacy Benefits Management

A pharmacy benefit manager (PBM) is a company that is under contract with managed care organizations, self-insured companies, and government programs to manage pharmacy network management, drug utilization review, outcomes management, and disease management. In simple terms, a PBM is a third-party administrator of prescription drug programs primarily responsible for processing and paying prescription drug claims. The PBM is also responsible for developing and maintaining the drug formulary, contracting with pharmacies, and negotiating discounts and rebates with drug manufacturers. As a pharmacist in this work setting, you may be called upon to create pharmacy benefit packages for employers or to fill drug prescriptions by mail order as part of a corporate health insurance plan.

Government Agencies

Local, state, and federal governmental agencies such as the National Institutes of Health (NIH), the FDA, the Center for Disease Control (CDC), the Department of Veterans Affairs (VA), and the Armed Forces require the expertise of skilled pharmacists to work in the hospitals and clinics in these agencies.

Again, chapter 16 covers all of the above career options within the pharmacy field in much greater detail.

COMPONENTS UNDER THE PHARMACY EDUCATION UMBRELLA

A pharmacy education is a foundation of knowledge around the central core of medications. This is very different from other healthcare providers; they are often focused on the diagnosis (physicians) and patient care (nursing). Pharmacy is an interdisciplinary field emphasizing the following six major areas of study:

- *Pharmacology* is an essential component in the study of pharmacy and deals with understanding the action of drugs in living systems. Pharmacology focuses on learning the effects of various doses of each drug and the different ways in which medicine can be introduced into the body. The study of toxicology examines the effects of poisons on living organisms and involves understanding the symptoms, mechanisms, treatments, and detection of poisoning.

- *Medicinal, or pharmaceutical, chemistry* is a scientific discipline at the intersection of chemistry and pharmacy involved with designing, synthesizing, and developing pharmaceutical drugs. Medicinal chemistry involves the identification, synthesis, and development of new chemical entities suitable for therapeutic use. This process is commonly referred to as drug discovery.

- *Pharmacognosy* is the study of medicines from natural sources (plants, animal-derived products, minerals). Most pharmacognostic studies are generally focused on medicinal plants/herbal medicines.

- *Business management* is commonly designated pharmacy administration. Instruction in this area of study includes the principles of basic economics, accounting, management, computer applications, and legal phases of the profession of pharmacy. These courses are especially helpful to graduates who plan to enter community pharmacy or to pharmacists who plan to become executives in pharmacies and/or hospitals.

- *Pharmacy practice* is designed to give students an appreciation of the background and nature of the profession. Instruction in pharmacy practice may include laboratory work to explore various scientific phenomena and the clinical application of the principles of pharmaceutical sciences. Essentially, pharmacy practice is the area within the pharmacy curriculum that deals with patient care and optimizing drug therapy.

- The *clinical, or experiential, component* of the pharmacy curriculum is designed to train students to become effective pharmacy practitioners; help develop students' communication skills for effective interaction with patients and other health professions; enable students to integrate and translate didactic learning into clinical practice; and help students develop a patient awareness in the practice of pharmacy and an awareness of their responsibility to provide optimal drug therapy.

In addition to the above six major disciplines, pharmacy also combines pharmaceutics, pharmacokinetics, pharmacodynamics, pharmacogenetics, pharmacogenomics, and pharmacovigilance into one profession:

- *Pharmaceutics* involves the design, development, and rational use of medications for the treatment and prevention of disease. It deals with understanding and improving drug delivery systems, how drug concentrations in the body can be optimized, the time course of drug action to determine the onset, duration of drug action, and side effects of particular medications in individual patients.

- *Pharmacokinetics* is the study of what the body does to a drug after a drug is ingested (how it gets absorbed in the body, breaks down and distributes, and finally gets eliminated from the body); whereas *pharmacodynamics* is the study of what a drug does to the body.

- *Pharmacogenetics* is the science of understanding the correlation between an individual patient's genetic makeup (genotype) and his or her response to drug treatment to ensure maximum efficacy with minimal adverse effects.

- *Pharmacogenomics* is the whole genome application of pharmacogenetics, which examines the single gene interactions with drugs. This discipline is sometimes referred to as "personalized medicine," in which drugs are optimized for each individual's unique genetic makeup with particular emphasis on improving drug safety.

- *Pharmacovigilance* is the science of collecting, monitoring, researching, assessing, and evaluating information from healthcare providers and patients on the adverse effects of medications in order to identify new information about hazards associated with medicine and, more importantly, to prevent harm to patients.

Pharmacy is a complex field of study that integrates many disciplines, with the ultimate goal of better understanding and optimizing the use of drugs in living systems. The broadness of the field is an attractive draw to the profession. Because various disciplines converge under one main pharmacy umbrella, a practicing pharmacist has many available career options to consider. This wide-ranging, all-encompassing aspect of the profession, coupled with the opportunity to help others every day, attracts pharmacists to the field.

CHAPTER 2

Making the Decision

The decision to become a pharmacist is a difficult one and should be evaluated carefully. Determining whether this career path is right for you can be a daunting task, but researching the field and asking the right questions can help you decide whether pharmacy is your ideal career choice. Your first step should be to get to know all about the profession and the time commitment required to achieve it. You also need to determine if you enjoy studying the sciences (biology, chemistry, math)—how do you feel about taking on an extremely challenging curriculum? Most importantly, you need to enjoy working with people and have the passion to help others. Above anything else, pharmacy is a people-oriented profession. This chapter will discuss the intricacies of a career in pharmacy so you can get a taste of the many lifestyle and career options available to you.

THE LIFE OF A PHARMACIST

Pharmacists, the highly-trained and skilled healthcare professionals who possess a Doctor of Pharmacy degree (PharmD), are drug therapy experts dedicated to optimizing medication management to produce positive health outcomes. Pharmacists are very knowledgeable on the chemical compositions of drugs and understand the effects they exhibit in the human body. Because they know how medications work and when and in what conditions to use them, pharmacists are often sought after for their advice on managing drug therapy. This is especially true for patients suffering from many health conditions that require multiple medications; a pharmacist is needed to ensure the multiple drug regimens are complementary to each other.

Ultimately, the pharmacist's principal goal is to help improve a patient's quality of life by optimizing therapy and ensuring the safe use of medication. You may have encountered the phrase "pharmaceutical care." The American Pharmacists Association (APhA) defines the principles of practice for someone offering pharmaceutical care as "a patient-centered, outcomes-oriented pharmacy practice that requires cooperation among the pharmacist, the patient, and other healthcare providers to achieve the following: to promote health, to prevent disease, and to assess, monitor, initiate, and optimize medication use to assure that drug therapy regimens are safe and effective."

The following sections list common pharmacist responsibilities.

Medication Distribution and Use

This is the job most people think of when a pharmacist comes to mind. Medication distribution and use involves processing prescriptions and dispensing drugs to patients. A pharmacist will also need to explain to the patient how the medication works, how to take the medication, the potential side effects, how best to store the medication, and what to do if a dose is missed.

Ensuring Drug Safety

Pharmacists have an important responsibility in monitoring the ongoing effectiveness and safety of medicines. As a member of the healthcare team, the pharmacist is a source of both information and critical evaluation of drug information. The pharmacist's expertise is vital to the application of the safety profile of a medicine to the needs of the patient. Thus, the pharmacist has a direct impact on the quality and safety of medication use. Pharmacist practitioners understand their pivotal role in the surveillance of the safe use of medicines through the early detection and reporting of suspected adverse drug events (ADEs) and other drug-related problems. In addition, the role of the pharmacist in post-marketing monitoring is not confined to ADEs and other drug-related problems reporting, but also in evaluating the safety of generics or therapeutically equivalent medicines and ensuring the proper use of complementary and alternative medicines as well as nonprescription over-the-counter medicines.

Medication Therapy Management (MTM)

Managing someone's health can become challenging and quite difficult if someone is taking more than one kind of medicine. This is especially true for the elderly population because they are often victims of multiple disease states and usually take a combination of different medications including over-the-counter drugs and herbal products. MTM is a comprehensive group of services provided by pharmacists as part of the Medicare Modernization Act of 2003 (which became effective in January 2006) to help patients get the most from the medications they are taking. MTM pharmacists work closely with patients and their doctors to solve any problems related to medication use, and to help patients get the best results from taking their medications. The practice of MTM was designed to improve patient care and to optimize medication use, which will eventually lead to improved patient outcomes.

MTM pharmacists are involved in managing and monitoring drug therapy in patients receiving treatments for cancer or chronic conditions (such as blood pressure control, asthma, or diabetes); consulting with patients on the proper use of drugs; performing and obtaining necessary assessments of patients' health status; formulating medication treatment plans; selecting, initiating, modifying, or administering drug therapy; and performing a comprehensive review to identify, resolve, and prevent any drug-related problems. In simple terms, an MTM pharmacist will help ensure that the patient is taking the right amount of medicine that he or she needs, that the drugs are not interacting with each other (especially with any vitamins or supplements), that the risk of adverse drug events is minimized and, most importantly, that the patient is receiving the right drug therapy and adequate care to manage his or her specific health condition. Specially trained MTM pharmacists will provide in-store medication reviews to identify problems or gaps in prescription drug therapy and then consult with the referring physician to recommend any specific changes in medication.

Disease State Management (DSM)

DSM is the process by which healthcare systems identify and treat and/or prevent diseases within defined patient populations. Pharmacists involved in DSM programs seek to manage and improve the health status of a carefully defined patient population over the entire course of a disease (such as diabetes or blood pressure control). Their work includes disease prevention efforts as well as patient management after the disease has developed.

Many community pharmacies have implemented DSM programs for managing diabetes, cholesterol, blood pressure, asthma, and similar health issues. For example, in diabetes management, the pharmacist would provide educational programs to patients about the disease, provide medication management and review, regularly monitor patients' self-tested and laboratory-tested blood glucose levels, educate patients on how to use their home blood glucose monitoring machines, monitor patients' compliance with drug therapies, and screen for any drug interactions or adverse drug events. The pharmacist also will consult with the referring physician to recommend any specific changes to the drug therapy.

Monitoring Patient Health Outcomes

A pharmacist needs to be able to recognize how a patient responds to drug therapy, then assess improvements in his or her patient's health outcome and quality of life, and, finally, adjust the therapy accordingly to achieve the original goals. The pharmacist works together with the healthcare team to monitor patient health outcomes as they relate to adequate drug therapy.

Providing Expert Advice to Healthcare Teams on Drug Decisions

As a drug expert, a pharmacist is expected to have a great bank of knowledge on different drug therapies. Pharmacists are often sought after by physicians, nurses, or other members of the healthcare team to provide the optimal drug therapy and the associated clinical studies to support their use for a particular condition.

Providing Drug Information to the Healthcare Team and Consumers

It cannot be emphasized enough that as a pharmacist you will not only need to know drug facts, but you also must be able to provide this knowledge to your colleagues and to consumers when asked about how a particular drug works. Pharmacists must be able to recommend over-the-counter or herbal products for treating common conditions such as colds or flu, pain relief, or local mild skin irritations. In addition, pharmacists also play an important role staffing poison control centers (PCCs) or poison information centers. PCCs receive calls from the general public and health professionals regarding exposures to poisonous or hazardous substances. These centers manage a 24-hour hotline and are continuously staffed by pharmacists, physicians, nurses, and poison information specialists who have received dedicated training in the field of toxicology. The specialist in poison information is a frontline provider who obtains the history of the exposure, assesses the toxicity risk, and determines the initial treatment for the patient. Thus, pharmacists provide clinical toxicology consultation to healthcare professionals who are treating exposed individuals.

Providing Expertise on Drug Composition and Drug Behavior

Pharmacists must understand the basic chemistry and pharmacology of drugs. Essentially, they should always be able to answer the following question: What is the chemical nature of this drug and how does the drug work once it is taken?

THE PROS AND CONS OF BEING A PHARMACIST

Pharmacy can be a very rewarding profession. You will enjoy interacting with a variety of individuals from patients to colleagues to other health professionals. You'll be responsible for ensuring your patients are getting optimal care in drug treatment, and you will be an integral part of the healthcare team. Even better, pharmacists tend to be both well paid and well respected. Here are some compelling reasons why you might consider pharmacy as a profession:

You Enjoy Helping People

Pharmacists are involved in improving the health of patients through reviewing medication profiles and optimizing drug usage, screening for drug allergies, and managing the side effects of drugs, among many other things. As a pharmacist, you are instrumental in helping people get well…which improves their quality of life.

> "The opportunity to truly help patients makes the profession of pharmacy so rewarding."
>
> —Tom, University of Maryland Pharmacy School

For example, you may notice that a patient is refilling her asthma medication (an inhaler that is prescribed by her doctor) more frequently than usual. Upon talking to the patient, she tells you that the inhaler is not helping her to control her breathing issues. You conduct a review of how she is using the inhaler to assess whether she is using the proper technique to allow optimal delivery of the drug to her lungs. In doing so, you find out that indeed the patient's inhaler technique was improper. You suggest that she participate in your pharmacy's asthma DSM program, which offers periodic review of her inhaler technique, ongoing monitoring of her lung function test to evaluate any breathing problems (using the peak-flow meter), and management of her medication use, such as encouraging compliance to drug regimens. A month later, the patient returns to the pharmacy for her routine refills and comments that she is doing much better and experiencing fewer breathing problems ever since she started using her inhaler properly. Because she feels better (due to your drug expertise), she is able to actively participate in other activities in her life.

Respect

Pharmacists have been regarded as the most accessible members of the healthcare team and are considered as some of the most trustworthy healthcare professionals. Because pharmacists are the experts on medicines and medication usage, patients and other healthcare professionals turn to them for this information and for advice on optimal drug therapy. Pharmacists are considered knowledgeable, honest, and caring—all attributes that contribute to the overall respect that pharmacists gain from the general public.

Flexibility

Careers in the pharmacy profession offer many options—with schedule as well as type of position. You can work full-time, part-time, or per diem (an individual who is hired to work on an as-needed basis and is paid by the day). Individuals with a family and young children can maintain a career as a pharmacist while raising a family.

For example, if you have to stay home with your children during the day while your spouse is at work, you may choose to practice pharmacy on weekends, during the night shift in a hospital pharmacy setting (which is always open), or at a 24-hour community pharmacy. Some hospital pharmacies offer 12-hour shifts, so you end up having a shorter 40-hour workweek. Pharmacy is so flexible that there is bound to be a schedule to accommodate your lifestyle. With the many options available, seeking balance between family and career is not as difficult a task.

Another advantage to pharmacy is that you can easily find a position throughout the country if you need to move. Because you are trained and equipped with a vast amount of medication knowledge, you can disseminate the fruits of your labor potentially in any pharmacy setting and location; therefore, you are not restricted to be at any particular place to practice your specialty.

Job Stability

Currently, because of the continuing shortage of pharmacists noted earlier, job prospects for pharmacists are very good. Professionals are in high demand and salaries continue to rise.

You Like a Challenge

As you can see from all of the information in this chapter, pharmacy is a very demanding and challenging position, with a tremendous amount of responsibility. First off, going to pharmacy school is a serious time and financial commitment. You will need to invest time in your education and you'll most likely be taking on a substantial financial burden until you graduate. Then, after you are a professional, your decisions and actions will affect individual patients' health and well-being; thus, you may also encounter the stress of being literally responsible for peoples' lives. Due to the existence of multiple medical problems every patient tends to have, coupled with being on multiple drug therapies, you must be particularly careful in screening for potentially life-threatening complications from drug interactions. It's a lot of pressure and a lot of work, and pharmacists must be up to the challenge on a day-to-day basis. In the end, however, it is quite rewarding to imagine the impact that you have on the lives of your patients who are now well because you took extra care to evaluate their medication profile, counsel them on the proper usage, and determine their effectiveness in treating the disease.

THE QUALITIES OF A PHARMACIST

As a pharmacist, you must possess certain desirable traits that will help you grow and become successful at what you do. To be an effective pharmacist, you must be attentive to details, hold high ethical standards, and maintain sound judgment and dependability while on the job. Sometimes being a pharmacist is like playing detective—you have to be extremely diligent in picking up the clues to a patient's medical and medication profile. Because many patients go to multiple specialists and often multiple drug stores, you'll need to investigate what medical problems the patient is suffering from and find out what other medications a patient is taking to prevent potentially life-threatening complications from drug interactions. You will need to be calm and collected if you are a pharmacist working at a Poison Control Center, because you will be fielding many phone calls that might be related to accidental childhood poisoning episodes.

Pharmacists, by law, are entrusted with the proper handling and dispensing of potentially dangerous and habit-forming substances. As such, you must be organized, maintain reliable records, and possess high ethical standards. Patients often look to you for advice and recommendations about their prescriptions, requiring you to play a vital role in helping them make decisions about their health, especially regarding issues with medication management. With the increasing number of products receiving FDA approval and becoming available on the market, you will need to stay up-to-date with current knowledge about these medications and be familiar with guidelines on their usage. Most importantly, you will need to possess excellent verbal skills to effectively communicate your knowledge to the patients and your colleagues on the healthcare team. After all, you are considered the medication expert, and people will look to you for your insight on optimal drug therapy.

The decision to join the pharmacy profession ultimately lies with you. If this is the right career for you, then you must be proactive in making the critical decisions that will help you achieve your goal.

PART TWO

Planning for Pharmacy School

CHAPTER 3

Planning Your Undergraduate Experience

Pharmacy school admissions committees look for well-rounded individuals who demonstrate a high level of scholastic achievement, maturity, personal motivation, and dedication in the serving of the community. Even if you're still in high school, it's never too early to prepare for pharmacy school.

DECIDING ON YOUR UNDERGRADUATE COLLEGE

The first step in planning for a pharmacy education is to plan your undergraduate education. While many pharmacy schools do not require a college degree, they do require that applicants fulfill the prepharmacy core requirements at an accredited college or university. With that said, prepharmacy students and their parents are often concerned with going to the "right" undergraduate school, one that will give the student the greatest chance of getting into pharmacy school. Although some pharmacy school admissions committees do consider the undergraduate institution attended when reviewing an applicant's academic history, you should not base your decision on selecting an undergraduate college on this factor. Keep in mind that it would be difficult for most pharmacy schools to agree upon the quality of education at any given undergraduate institution let alone provide you with the rankings of undergraduate schools. Therefore, a better way to approach the issue of which undergraduate college to attend is to compile a list of schools you believe will enable you to do your best work. Some factors to consider include classroom size, location and convenience to home, quarter versus semester system, and undergraduate programs offered.

Remember, college should be a time of development—from emotional, spiritual, physical, and intellectual perspectives. The years that you spend as an undergraduate are some of the most important in your life. Most individuals after graduating from college agree that getting the complete undergraduate experience helped to develop their maturity, goals, and knowledge as well as better prepare them for the real-world work environment.

Two-Year Versus Four-Year Colleges

Many potential applicants wonder if they can complete part of their undergraduate education at a two-year community college and whether this will make their application less competitive than an applicant who attends a four-year college. While you may take some courses at a two-year school, whenever possible, you should complete your prerequisite science courses at a four-year institution. Many admissions committees look to your performance in undergraduate science courses as being a good predictor of your potential to handle the pharmacy school curriculum. Always strive to perform well in the most academically challenging environment available to you, which typically means completing the prepharmacy coursework at a four-year college. In addition, many admissions committees may not consider grades earned from community colleges when evaluating your science grade point average (GPA). Be sure to check with each pharmacy school you're applying to on their specific requirements for completing prerequisites and what courses are acceptable and count toward your science GPA.

Once you've decided on the undergraduate college of your choice, the following timetable is a useful guide to help you plan ahead, starting from the first year of your college career. As you can see, this timetable is intended for those students who choose to attend a four-year college. It highlights what you should try to accomplish each year. Further details to each bulleted point are provided later in this chapter.

YEAR IN COLLEGE*	WHAT YOU SHOULD TRY TO ACCOMPLISH
Freshman	• Begin taking your prerequisite courses for pharmacy. • Concentrate on your studies. • Get involved in student organizations. • Visit your college career center and find out if your school has a prepharmacy student society. Sign up to receive information regarding pharmacy-related events, workshops, professional events, etc. • Research the field of pharmacy.
Sophomore	• Talk to practicing pharmacists. • Get some experience in a pharmacy-related setting. • Research different pharmacy programs. Visit pharmacy schools' websites and find out about their prepharmacy requirements (whether you need to take the Pharmacy College Admission Test [PCAT] at this time). • Participate in information sessions or campus tours that are offered at the pharmacy schools you find compelling.
Junior	• Request the pharmacy schools' applications and keep a careful eye on deadlines. • Take the PCAT. (See chapter 4 for more on this test.) • Begin requesting letters of recommendation and writing your personal statement. • Participate in career center workshops related to applying to professional school.
Senior	• Submit your pharmacy school applications. • Prepare for your interviews. • Apply for financial assistance. • Complete your prepharmacy requirements.

*Please note that many programs accept students after two years of undergraduate preparation. If you choose to follow this route, your timeline will be compressed.

CHOOSING AN UNDERGRADUATE MAJOR

While a bachelor's degree is not required for pharmacy school, all applicants are required to complete certain prepharmacy course requirements at an accredited college or university. Most schools accept students into their pharmacy programs once they've completed at least two years of undergraduate study, however, in recent years, there has been a growing trend of successful applicants who hold a bachelor's degree. As such, most pharmacy programs now highly recommend a four-year program with an increasing number of applicants who will receive a bachelor's degree by the time they attend pharmacy school.

In general, admissions committees look for well-rounded candidates with a proficiency in the sciences. Therefore, as long as you demonstrate your academic ability in the sciences by doing well in the required prepharmacy core science courses, you should choose an undergraduate major that interests you the most. Remember, you will most likely get better grades if you study a field in which you really enjoy investing time. With that said, while many pharmacy applicants are science majors (chemistry, biology, etc.), pharmacy students come from a wide variety of educational backgrounds with majors as diverse as English, business, economics, social sciences, and the like.

While we have emphasized that you should choose a major that interests you the most, we also understand that this could be a difficult choice to make. There are many advantages and disadvantages to weigh in your decision.

Science majors often have a significant academic advantage in pharmacy school over their classmates who did not major in science. This is because the first two years of pharmacy school curriculum cover the basic sciences (biochemistry, microbiology, physiology) and science majors are more likely to have studied some of these subjects in detail during their upper-division coursework. Thus, these science majors often find the first two years of pharmacy school less demanding. Another benefit of majoring in the sciences is that you will most likely fulfill much of your pharmacy prerequisites simply by completing your major requirements. One disadvantage for science majors who have taken the minimum of nonscience courses may be that many admissions committees look for applicants with demonstrated interests in the world around them as exemplified by a broad selection of the courses they take.

If your major is in a nonscience field, then your work in both science and nonscience courses will be evaluated. However, with fewer courses on which to judge your science ability, your grades in the core science courses will have greater importance. This does not mean that nonscience majors are at a disadvantage compared to science majors. The more important basis for admission to pharmacy school is your undergraduate transcript, no matter what your major is. Remember, if you enjoy what you are studying and majoring in, this is usually reflected with a strong transcript. If you thoroughly enjoy and excel in a particular area (in addition to the sciences), always choose the major that fits your interest. Your grades will thank you for this decision.

PREPHARMACY COURSE REQUIREMENTS

The pharmacy curriculum reflects a broad, multidisciplinary science base. The science in pharmacy is focused on three broad fields: mathematics, physical sciences, and biology. Therefore, adequate preparation in these courses is mandatory because they are the fundamental basic sciences that are essential to the pharmacy curriculum. These courses promote the development of a student's critical thinking and problem-solving skills. The basic coursework requirements of pharmacy programs follow.

Mathematics

(at least calculus level)

Mathematics is important because pharmacists use a lot of math when dispensing prescriptions—determining proper drug dosage levels, preparing formulas of many types, and configuring certain chemical calculations. You will need to learn the various weights and measures used in pharmacy to calculate doses of drugs given to people of different ages and weights. Pharmacists also are expected to know how to figure out the amount of material to use for certain chemical solutions and many other pharmaceutical calculations.

Physical Sciences

(one year of general chemistry plus lab, one year of organic chemistry plus lab, and one year of physics plus lab)

Instruction in the physical sciences is required because the principles are basic to many pharmaceutical practices. Physics and chemistry are interrelated disciplines, as both are needed to understand the behavior and properties of drugs and matter. The fineness of powdered drugs, the transfer of heat, the behavior of gases, and the formation and decay of radioactive isotope (in nuclear pharmacy) are all based on a thorough understanding of both disciplines. Pharmacists deal with many medical substances that are pure chemicals. Thus, you must learn how to properly handle and store them, how to analyze them to determine their purity, and how to dissolve them, combine them, package them, and preserve them. You will need to know the principles of basic chemistry as they are applied in the study of medicinal products.

Biological Sciences

(biology, anatomy, physiology, microbiology, and biochemistry)

Many drugs are derived from plants and animals. The study of biological sciences is necessary for building a strong foundation of knowledge of natural drugs and their actions within the body. Instruction in the biological sciences will also enable students to understand the mechanisms of how drugs work in the body and how the body breaks down these entities.

Nonscience Courses

In addition, classes in English composition and communication/speech, as well as electives in humanities and social and behavioral sciences will help you understand and communicate with people, thereby enabling you to practice more effectively within society. These courses are designed to enhance your people skills, an element that is essential to the idea of pharmacy as a "people profession."

Sample Requirements Timeline

Here is a sample outline of how you should try to pace the completion of your prerequisite coursework over four years of undergraduate study:

Freshman year.

Many applicants complete the one-year general chemistry (with the associated laboratory class) requirement during their first year. Other prerequisites to consider include lower-division biology, math, English, and other lower-division courses required for your major.

Sophomore year.

During the second year, many students complete the one-year organic chemistry requirement, lower-division biology, and other lower-division courses required for their major. Some students may also be able to complete or at least start on their physics requirements during this time.

Junior year.

Many applicants often complete the one-year physics requirement during this year and any electives or upper-division courses required for their major.

Senior year.

By now, most students have completed all the prerequisites for pharmacy school and any requirements or electives for their major. (Note: If you have not finished all your prepharmacy requirements, remember that this coursework must be completed by the summer before you are to begin your pharmacy education.)

Consult Your PSAR

The best source for specific information on prerequisites is the Pharmacy School Admission Requirements, also known as the PSAR. Published every year by the Association of American Colleges of Pharmacy (AACP), it provides comprehensive information on all the pharmacy schools in the United States. The PSAR profiles the pharmacy schools and includes tables detailing applicant profiles, requirements, programs offered, deadlines, and tuition. A copy of this publication can be purchased from the AACP (please refer to the AACP website for more information at www.aacp.org). However, it is very important that throughout your college career you contact your schools of interest for their prepharmacy course requirements and the most up-to-date information.

Completion of all prepharmacy requirements provides essential preparation for the rigorous four-year professional curriculum in pharmacy school. While these requirements may be completed at any accredited two-year or four-year college or university, it is again recommended that you complete the prerequisite science courses at a four-year institution. All courses must be completed with letter grades of C or higher—grades on a pass/no-pass system are usually not accepted. Most pharmacy colleges require a minimum GPA of a 3.0 (or a B average) during the first two years. Always strive to maintain your GPA as high as possible. If you are approaching advanced sciences where the subject matter may be getting difficult, try your best to work hard and get through the course with as high a grade as possible. Complex sciences are going to be tough at first (especially if the subject matter is completely new to you), but the work usually gets a little easier as you become more familiar with the subject material. Even an upward trend in grade performance will be viewed in a positive light, especially when you are trying to overcome a less than spectacular year.

Advanced Placement Examination Credit

If you knew in high school that you had an interest in the sciences, you might already have received high school advanced placement (AP) credit for lower-division courses. For many students (depending on the undergraduate institution you attend), this means that you do not have to retake those particular courses. While AP credit may satisfy certain pharmacy prerequisite requirements, you'll want to make sure (early on in your undergraduate career) that your pharmacy schools of choice will accept your AP credits. This is an institutional decision; therefore, if you have received high school AP credit, contact each school you're applying to regarding its institutional policy.

THE OPTION OF ONLINE CLASSES

Given today's advancement in information technology and the availability of distance learning, online coursework may be a tempting option. While online courses allow a lot of flexibility with regards to time and geographic location, one disadvantage of this type of learning involves the lack of direct interaction with the instructor or the hands-on experience that is gained from a classroom setting. If you are a visual learner and thrive from face-to-face interaction with the professor and your classmates, you may not do well without that interaction. In this situation, as tempting as at-home learning may be, the online format would not be a suitable option. More importantly, credits from your online coursework may be difficult to transfer. In general, this format of learning is usually not accepted in place of prerequisites taken in the traditional classroom setting. Before applying, be sure to contact your schools of choice to inquire about whether online coursework will transfer.

Most pharmacy schools do not specify that you need to finish all of your prerequisites before submitting your application. However, some schools prefer that you complete a certain percentage of them, and some have requirements for the number that must be taken for a grade. Consult the PSAR on the policies of the different schools to which you want to apply. Keep in mind that completion of your prepharmacy coursework is required prior to beginning your pharmacy curriculum. Therefore, it is imperative that you keep each pharmacy admission office updated on the completion of your requirements throughout your application process.

EXTRACURRICULAR ACTIVITIES

In addition to intellectual and academic competence, pharmacy school admissions committees also evaluate your nonacademic qualities, such as your commitment to community service, your pharmacy-related or healthcare-related experience, and your overall motivation for pursuing a career in pharmacy. The pharmacy profession requires strong people skills, and extracurricular activities will not only be interesting and informative, but will also showcase your ability to work well with others of diverse backgrounds. It doesn't matter if these are science-related. The point is to get you out there in your school community, challenging your body and mind even when you are not in the classroom. Pursuing extracurricular activities that interest you and that can exemplify your leadership and communication skills will make you an attractive candidate for any admissions committee.

Pharmacy schools select applicants who will become future leaders in the profession. Your participation in campus or community organizations, sports, and clubs—especially any leadership positions—is a great way to acquire leadership skills. Your involvement in community service not only demonstrates your interest and willingness to help people, but can also help you develop interpersonal communication skills.

ON-THE-JOB EXPERIENCE

Gaining pharmacy-related experience is invaluable because it demonstrates your understanding of (and interest in) the profession. While it is impossible to gain experience as an actual pharmacist, you may gain exposure to pharmacy by setting up a volunteer or shadow experience in a pharmacy-related setting (e.g., a hospital pharmacy, community pharmacy, or retail pharmacy). Find out from your college guidance counselor or the career center about volunteer opportunities. If your undergraduate college is located near the university's medical center, the opportunity to volunteer at a hospital pharmacy is right there in your backyard. Contacting the hospital's volunteer program is the best first step. You may also find pharmacy-related opportunities through networking from any prepharmacy professional organization sponsored at your college or university. This student group usually hosts different events at its meetings. It may offer such opportunities as a session where you are able to meet practicing pharmacists in the community who speak about their experiences. You may also try going to your local independent pharmacy and talking to the pharmacist there about shadowing him or her. Gaining this experience will help you explore the real-life day-to-day of pharmacy. Take the opportunity to learn about the pharmacy profession and find out whether this career path is the right choice for you.

You may also consider volunteering in different pharmacy environments to get a broader perspective of the various kinds of pharmacy settings. For example, you can spend one summer at a local community pharmacy and the next summer at a hospital pharmacy. Other healthcare-related experiences may include volunteering at a hospital or in a research laboratory. While research experience is not required for pharmacy school admission, developing research skills will be beneficial if you have a strong interest in seeking a future research or academic career in pharmacy.

Your extracurricular activities can be highlighted in different ways throughout the application process. Aside from listing all of the activities on your application, you may choose to discuss some of them in your personal statement or in your short essay responses in the supplemental application to the Pharmacy College Application Service (PharmCAS). (Refer to chapter 8 for a discussion of the PharmCAS, an online application method for many pharmacy schools.) You will also have a chance to describe your experiences in detail during your school interview. Remember, a well-rounded person who takes the time to interact with the community is just as impressive as one with stellar marks on paper.

Quick Tips for Prepharmacy Students

- Major in a field that interests you the most.
- Maintain good grades.
- Explore the field of pharmacy.
- Get some real-world experience in a pharmacy-related setting.
- Demonstrate your leadership and communication abilities through extracurricular activities.

CHAPTER 4

The Pharmacy College Admission Test (PCAT)

The Pharmacy College Admission Test (PCAT) is an exam developed by The Psychological Corporation, a brand of Pearson. It is a specialized test that helps identify qualified applicants to pharmacy colleges by measuring the general academic ability and scientific knowledge necessary to succeed in a pharmacy education. The American Assoication of Colleges and Pharmacy (AACP) endorses the PCAT as the official preferred admission test for entrance to pharmacy school. While the exam is designed specifically for this purpose, it is not an admissions requirement for all schools. You will need to inquire from the schools you're interested in applying to whether the PCAT is an admissions requirement for their program. This information can be found on the AACP website at www.aacp.org, or you can contact PCAT directly at 800-622-3231.

WHAT'S ON THE TEST

The PCAT consists of seven timed sections: 240 multiple-choice qestions in Verbal Ability, Biology, Reading Comprehension, Quantitative Ability, Chemistry, and two Writing sections. Candidates are given four hours to complete the exam and time for one short break halfway through the exam.

The total test breakdown as you will see it on test day is as follows:

Writing (Essay 1)

Time: 30 minutes

Format: Problem-solving essay based on a given topic

What it tests: General composition skills and conventions of language, ability to communicate a solution to a problem

Verbal Ability

Time: 30 minutes

Format: 48 multiple-choice questions

What it tests: General, nonscientific word knowledge using analogies and sentence completion

Biology

Time: 30 minutes

Format: 48 multiple-choice questions

What it tests: Knowledge of the concepts and principles of basic biology with an emphasis on human biology, microbiology, and anatomy/physiology

Chemistry

Time: 30 minutes

Format: 48 multiple-choice questions

What it tests: Knowledge of the concepts and principles of inorganic and elementary organic chemistry

Writing (Essay 2)

Time: 30 minutes

Format: Problem-solving essay based on a given topic

What it tests: General composition skills and conventions of language, ability to communicate a solution to a problem

Reading Comprehension

Time: 50 minutes

Format: 48 multiple-choice questions; there are 6 passages with 6–9 questions about each

What it tests: Ability of the student to comprehend, analyze, and interpret reading passages on scientific topics

Quantitative Ability

Time: 40 minutes

Format: 48 multiple-choice questions

What it tests: Skills in arithmetic processes, including fractions, decimals, and percents, and the ability to reason through and understand quantitative concepts and their relationships, including applications of algebra, probability and statistics, pre-calculus, and calculus

HOW THE PCAT IS SCORED

Each PCAT section receives its own score. Each section is scored on a scale ranging from 200–600, with 600 as the highest and a mean of 400.

The Writing section is scored numerically from 0 to 5. One of the Writing prompts will be experimental and will not count toward your score. Two Writing scores will be recorded: one reflecting use of appropriate grammar and style and the other reflecting ability to create and support a solution to a problem.

The number of multiple-choice questions that you answer correctly per section is your "raw score." Your raw score will then be converted to yield the "scaled score"—the one that will fall somewhere in that 200–600 range. These scaled scores are reported to pharmacy schools as your PCAT scores. All multiple-choice questions are worth the same amount—one raw point—so there's no penalty for guessing. That means that you should always fill in an answer for every question, whether you get to that question or not! Never let time run out on any section without filling in an answer for every question on the grid. Your score report will tell you—and your potential pharmacy schools—not only your scaled scores, but also the national mean score for each section, as well as standard deviations, national scoring profiles for each section, and your percentile ranking.

Your Percentile

The percentile figure tells you how many other test-takers scored at or below your level. In other words, a percentile figure of 80 means that 80 percent did as well or worse than you did and that only 20 percent did better.

You should receive your scores in the mail approximately four to five weeks after taking the exam. The schools that you indicated on your initial application will also receive an official score report. Your most recent PCAT score as well as any PCAT scores that you earned in the past five years will be reported on the official score report sent to the institution unless you selected the "No Score Option" at the time of testing. Scores more than five years old will not be reported.

What's a Good Score?

There's no such thing as a cut-and-dried good score. Much depends on the strength of the rest of your application (if your transcript is first-rate, the pressure to excel on the PCAT isn't as intense) and on where you want to go to school (different schools have different score expectations). For each PCAT administration, the average scaled scores are approximately 400 for each section; this equates to the 50th percentile. You need scores of at least 450 to be considered competitive by most pharmacy schools, and if you're aiming for the top schools, you must do even better and score above 450.

It's important to maximize your performance on every question. Just a few questions one way or the other can make a big difference in your scaled score. You should make an extra effort to score well on a test section if you did poorly in a corresponding class. So the best revenge for getting a C in chemistry class is acing the Chemistry section of the PCAT.

PCAT COMPUTER-BASED TESTING

Beginning in July 2011, all candidates will take the PCAT via the computer. Be assured that the new computer-based test (CBT) version of the PCAT is exactly the same as the paper-and-pencil form in terms of content, order of subtests, scoring, and reporting. The only difference is in the way the test is administered. You will be required to type your essay responses for the CBT version.

TIPS FOR TAKING THE PCAT

The following strategies are suggested to help you do your best on the PCAT:

- Familiarize yourself with the test by reviewing the test components thoroughly.
- Consider enrolling in a PCAT prep course.
- Be prepared physically and mentally. Because most of the test involves knowledge, skills, and abilities accumulated over time, cramming probably will not help much.
- Answer all multiple-choice questions—even if you have to guess. Every PCAT question is worth a single point regardless of the degree of difficulty. If you can't answer a question or can't get to it because you've run out of time, then guess. Remember, there is no penalty for guessing, so it is to your advantage to answer every question.
- Do not dwell on items that are unfamiliar or difficult. Because all the multiple-choice items count the same, skip around and answer the easy questions first and return to the difficult ones later if time permits. Do not leave any question unanswered. Fill in an answer to every question on the test whether you have time to get to it or not.

> **Be a Control Freak**
>
> The PCAT should be viewed just like any other part of your application: as an opportunity to show the pharmacy schools who you are and what you can do.
>
> Take control of your PCAT experience.

- Learn a step-by-step approach to the writing sample.
- Be sure to remain calm during the test. If you've encountered a difficult passage, don't get upset about it and let it throw off your performance on the rest of the section. Most likely, you won't be the only one having trouble with it. Just remember to stay focused and move on to the next set of questions.
- Always keep track of time and pace yourself. Do not spend a disproportionate amount of time on any one question or group of questions. Allow ample time at the end of each section to fill in answers for any questions you've skipped or haven't gotten to yet.

- Practice, practice, practice! Take all of the PCAT practice tests you can. The more you practice, the more comfortable and confident you will be with the exam.

TEST DATES AND REGISTRATION

Talk to your prepharmacy advisor to find out about the latest PCAT administration schedule and how to register for the test. If you don't have an advisor, contact the PCAT Program Office. They'll send you a registration packet that contains important information on PCAT fees and score reporting.

To check for test dates and deadlines, visit the PCAT website at *www.pcatweb.info* for current information. It is wise to apply early because test centers have limited seating and assign seats on a first-come, first-serve basis. In addition, your desired testing location could fill to capacity soon after PCAT registration begins and not be available, especially if you are applying close to a deadline.

> ### Plan Ahead
> The PCAT is offered only a few times a year, so be sure to give yourself lots of lead time for getting information. Download a PCAT Candidate Information Booklet at www.pcatweb.info.

More than 98 percent of applicants register online to take the PCAT. Applications for the PCAT must be received no later than six weeks prior to the scheduled test date. You may also apply online between the Standard Registration Deadline and the Late Registration Deadline (two weeks before the test date); however, this requires a $49 late fee in addition to the $150 online application fee (for the 2010–2011 test dates). Note that late registration is possible only if completed online. For detailed registration information, visit the PCAT website.

CHAPTER 5

Selecting the Right Program

As of Fall 2001, all accredited pharmacy schools no longer offer a bachelor of science degree in pharmacy. The Doctor of Pharmacy degree (PharmD) is now the sole professional degree, which generally requires four academic years of study after your undergraduate education. Pharmacy programs used to award two professional degrees: the Bachelor of Science in Pharmacy (BS Pharm) and the Doctor of Pharmacy (PharmD). The bachelor's degree required five years of collegiate study, whereas the PharmD is a four-year program following a minimum of two years of prepharmacy coursework. But as the pharmacy profession continues to change, so does the education of pharmacists. The main level of pharmacy education has advanced to the entry-level, clinically based PharmD degree, replacing the BS Pharm degree. This transition occurred to better prepare pharmacists for the growing importance of clinical roles in the field.

There are many different types of pharmacy school programs that you may consider applying to. In general, all schools offer the traditional professional (four-year) program, and some also offer the other types of unique programs we will discuss in this chapter. Applying to a pharmacy school program should be a well-researched decision. Each of the schools in the United States is different and can offer you a unique experience. Before you start filling out applications, you need to take the time to decide what kind of experience you hope to get during your four years of study. Doing so will better equip you with the knowledge you need to narrow down potential programs into a final list from which you will ultimately choose the right program for yourself.

TRADITIONAL PHARMD PROGRAMS

The majority of programs accept students into the professional pharmacy degree program upon completion of the pharmacy course prerequisites. While most students enter pharmacy school with three or more years of undergraduate college experience, some pharmacy programs require or give preference to applicants who have previously earned a bachelor's (BS/BA) degree. Regardless of the educational background of the entering pharmacy student, all individuals must complete the full four academic years (or three calendar years) of pharmacy study.

There are several factors to consider when deciding which pharmacy program is right for you, and they will be discussed in the next sections.

How Do You Want to Spend Your Four Years?

Each pharmacy school allots its four-year study plan in a different way. The first three years of pharmacy school usually cover *didactic learning*. This is pharmacy coursework based in the classroom setting. The last year usually involves the *experiential training*, which is the clinical component of the curriculum (also referred to as "clerkships" or "rotations"), where pharmacy students will participate in structured and supervised training to learn about the practice of pharmacy.

> "I enjoyed my pharmacy education; however, I found the clinical rotation to be the highlight. Rounding on the wards with the medical team and having an impact on the patient's pharmacotherapy was gratifying."
>
> —Amy, pharmacy student, University of Colorado

These advanced pharmacy practice experiences help students acquire practice skills and develop the level of confidence and responsibility necessary for entry into the profession as a pharmacist. The various practice sites represent the range of opportunities available to pharmacists. At the sites, students are trained by licensed pharmacists (known as "preceptors"), who help students understand how to apply classroom learning to daily practice, facilitating their transition from a pharmacy student to a practicing pharmacist. Some pharmacy schools also offer introductory pharmacy practice experiences (referred to as "externships") earlier on in the curriculum as a means to introduce students to the basic practice of pharmacy.

There are other options, too. Some schools may have their students begin an advanced pharmacy practice experience a semester earlier than most PharmD programs, thereby lengthening their experience training to enhance the pharmacy practice component. Yet other programs offer a **pathway-specific** approach, presenting the opportunity for students to concentrate on a particular discipline within pharmacy, such as in pharmaceutical care, research, or health policy and management.

> "I'm glad I chose a research-intensive university. I'm now leaning toward doing a PhD in pharmaceutics."
>
> —Erika, pharmacy student, University of Minnesota

Before adding a pharmacy school to your list, find out how its students spend their time there and think about what you want out of your pharmacy school experience. Are you more interested in research and would thus prefer to attend a research-intensive school? Maybe you'd rather spend your time in pharmacy practice and therefore would prefer a program with a strong clinical component or more training in the advance pharmacy practice experience clerkships? Do you function better in a quarter versus a semester system? Even if other aspects of a school are compelling, focus on what you'll be doing with the bulk of your time before committing to an application.

The Top 25 Research-Intensive Pharmacy Institutions

Ohio State University
Purdue University
University at Buffalo—State University
   of New York
University of Arizona
University of California—San Diego
University of California—San Francisco
University of Colorado
University of Florida
University of Illinois—Chicago
University of Iowa
University of Kansas
University of Kentucky
University of Maryland

University of Michigan
University of Minnesota
University of Mississippi
University of North Carolina—
   Chapel Hill
University of Pittsburgh
University of Southern California
University of Tennessee
University of Texas
University of Utah
University of Washington
University of Wisconsin—Madison
Virginia Commonwealth University

How Many Years Do You Want to Spend in a Pharmacy Program?

As stated above, the typical program is four years. However, careful research may find you a few pharmacy schools that offer alternate options.

Three-year accelerated programs.

A small number of pharmacy institutions offer a year-round PharmD degree program to students who have completed all college-level prerequisites for admission. This accelerated program gives students an opportunity to complete their PharmD in three calendar years by completing the pharmacy curriculum full-time, year-round, with no summer breaks as opposed to the traditional four-year program, which offers summer breaks. Contact the schools directly to inquire about such programs.

"0-6" programs or six-year professional degree programs for high school students.

You may even be able to get an early start on your pharmacy education. There are a few pharmacy schools that accept students directly from high school. These are referred to as "0-6" programs because they allow students to complete their prepharmacy and professional study within six years after high school graduation. Students enrolled in a "0-6" program who successfully complete the first two years of preprofessional study (and any other stated contingencies) are guaranteed admission into the four-year professional pharmacy degree program. So if you know for certain that you want a career in pharmacy before entering college, then you might consider the six-year program leading to the PharmD degree. This is considered a fast-track approach to getting your professional pharmacy degree and is best suited for individuals who are bright, highly motivated, and determined to complete their pharmacy degree in the shortest amount of time possible.

However, given the expanding complexity in the role of today's pharmacists, more students enter pharmacy school with three or more years of undergraduate coursework. As we've previously mentioned, it is increasingly common for pharmacy schools to give preference to students holding a bachelor's degree. Most pharmacy school admissions committees find that students who complete an undergraduate degree are better prepared to handle the demanding pharmacy curriculum. In addition, many students feel that taking the time to complete four years of undergraduate study allows them a chance to explore other career options and assess whether pharmacy is the right career path for them. College graduates agree that the undergraduate experience is an important period in their lives that fosters growth and maturity as an individual and a professional.

"Early Assurance" programs.

In addition to "0-6" programs, there are a few pharmacy schools that offer "early assurance" (also known as "early admission") status for selected high school students. As with "0-6" programs, students who enroll in an "early assurance" program must successfully complete the first two years of preprofessional study to be guaranteed admission into the four-year professional pharmacy program. These programs are not categorized as "0-6" because the majority of students enrolled are admitted as "transfer" students after completion of at least two years of college. You will need to contact colleges and schools directly to determine if they have an "early assurance" program available to high school students.

What Is Your Classroom Size Preference?

Classroom size is dependent upon the faculty-to-student ratio. Some schools admit a larger number of students than other schools. If you are a student who learns better in a smaller classroom size, then pay special attention to the number of applicants admitted to the particular school and find out the faculty-to-student ratio.

LOCATION

If location is an important factor in terms of your decision-making process, then find out how many schools with programs that interest you are present in the city or state in which you would want to live. Because the experiential component, or clinical rotation, is a part of the overall pharmacy school curriculum, you will also need to determine where the potential clerkship sites where you will be doing your rotations are. Clerkships are usually offered at a variety of pharmacy practice settings and include hospitals, clinics, retail pharmacy chains, independent pharmacies, drug information centers, pharmaceutical companies, government agencies, or managed care organizations. Contact each school for information regarding the types and location of clerkship sites offered through its program. This information will help you estimate your travel time for commuting between the actual school itself and the potential clerkship sites. Because some schools may be based far from major medical centers, you may be required to temporarily relocate during this rotation period so that you can complete the required clerkship. This is information you should inquire about before you start any program.

Housing

Remember that in addition to tuition, you'll also have to pay for housing, food, and transportation. Unfortunately, due to the location of some schools, nearby housing is either unsafe or unaffordable. In

> **Read All about It**
>
> If you're considering a particular locale, get your hands on its local newspaper. This will give you an idea of the cost of living, available transportation, and community issues.

some inner-city schools, the majority of the student body resides in dormitories. These dorms are often expensive and have inadequate kitchen facilities. Nonetheless, they may be the best alternative given the pharmacy school's location.

In contrast, students who decide to attend equally good programs that are based in small towns may be pleasantly surprised to find inexpensive housing near the school.

COST

Pharmacy school is a substantial financial commitment. Although student loans and scholarships are available, you should find out the cost of tuition so that you can determine what kind and how much of financial assistance you will need to apply for. Tuition varies for each pharmacy school and is determined by whether the institution is private or public and your state of residency (in-state versus out-of-state residents). Keep in mind that the difference in cost between attending a state and a private pharmacy school can be striking. When figuring out the actual cost of attending a pharmacy school, remember to take account of all factors, including tuition, fees, and cost of living (room, board, etc.). Part Five of this book goes into detail about how you can make the costs of pharmacy school work for you and your family.

ACCREDITATION

It is essential that the pharmacy school you attend meets the standards established by the Accreditation Council for Pharmacy Education (ACPE), the body that is responsible for accrediting PharmD-granting programs in the United States. The Board of Directors of the ACPE is made up of representatives appointed by the American Association of Colleges of Pharmacy (AACP), the American Pharmacists Association (APhA), the National Association of Boards of Pharmacy (NABP), the American Council on Education (ACE), as well as representatives of the general public.

The ACPE is the sole accreditation agency recognized by the U.S. Department of Education to accredit professional degree programs in pharmacy. For the directory of accredited pharmacy school programs or to determine the accreditation status for a particular institution, contact the ACPE directly:

Accreditation Council for Pharmacy Education
20 N. Clark Street
Suite 2500
Chicago, IL 60602-5109
Phone: (312) 664-3575
www.acpe-accredit.org

Because of the recent emergence of newly established pharmacy degree programs, there are different types of accreditation status. A new pharmacy school program may be granted one of two preaccreditation statuses—**precandidate or candidate**—which depend upon its stage of development, and usually progresses through both statuses.

Precandidate

A new program that has no students enrolled, but has a dean, may be granted precandidate status. This means that the planning of the program has taken into account ACPE standards and suggests reasonable assurances of moving to the next step of candidate status.

Candidate

A new program that has students enrolled but has not had a graduating class may be granted candidate status, indicating it is a developmental program. This means the program has taken into account ACPE standards and is expected to mature in accordance to stated plans within a defined time period and with reasonable assurances that the program will become accredited as programmatic experience is gained, generally by the time the first class has been graduated. Graduates of a "candidate status" class have the same rights and privileges as graduates of a fully accredited program.

The decision of whether to enroll in a new pharmacy school should be carefully made. Pharmacy institutions are not eligible to be granted accreditation status until they have graduated their first PharmD class. Thus, students who attend a new pharmacy degree program may be taking a risk if the institution does not receive full accreditation status at that time. Graduates from unaccredited pharmacy schools are ineligible to sit for the state pharmacy license examination or practice pharmacy in the United States.

BALANCING PERSONAL AND ACADEMIC LIFE

While academics remain a high priority, an important issue that applicants should take into consideration is the ability to balance personal life with academic life. This factor is especially critical to students with children, spouses, or other individuals to whom they are responsible. Pharmacy schools vary widely in the demands and intensity of their curricula outside the classroom, as well as the social culture of the school and student body. You should research each potential pharmacy school of interest and talk to current and former pharmacy students to learn the crucial details that will affect your life, not just your academic career.

Pharmacy Institutions with Religious Affiliations

Belmont University—Christian
Creighton University—Jesuit—Catholic
Duquesne University Mylan School of Pharmacy, Spiritan—Catholic
Harding University—Christian
Lipscomb University—Christian
Loma Linda University—Christian
Ohio Northern University—United Methodist
Presbyterian College—Presbyterian
Regis University—Jesuit Catholic
Saint Joseph College—Catholic
Samford University—Baptist
Saint John Fisher College—Catholic
Saint John's University—Catholic
Shenandoah University—United Methodist Church
Touro College—Jewish
Touro University—Jewish
Union University—Christian
University of the Incarnate Word—Catholic
Wingate University—Judeo-Christian
Xavier University of Louisiana—Catholic

ALTERNATIVE PHARMACY SCHOOL PROGRAMS

In addition to the traditional four-year, classroom-based pharmacy school programs, there are other options that you may find match better with your lifestyle.

Distance Learning Programs or Online Programs

Some pharmacy colleges and schools currently offer distance learning programs that are web-based and designed primarily for practicing pharmacists with a BS degree in pharmacy who wish to return to school to earn a PharmD degree so they may enhance their skills. Other pharmacy degree programs may offer satellite campus options or part-time degree programs. Creighton University is the only institution to offer an online program for entry-level candidates. Creighton University offers the first and only accredited Doctor of Pharmacy Program Distance Pathway (Online Pharmacy Program) providing a full-time educational method to obtain a PharmD degree. This online program covers the same material as the traditional on-campus pathway, but allows students to take didactic coursework using distance mechanisms (e.g., the Internet and CD-ROMs) from wherever they live. Students are able to interact with faculty and mentors via Internet chat rooms, email, fax, and telephone. The didactic portion of the distance pathway is taught on a semester basis with students completing the on-campus laboratory courses in a condensed manner during the summers and lasting for one to two weeks. The clinical component of the online pharmacy program requires eight five-week clinical rotations. Sites for the clinical rotations are in a variety of locations throughout the country and include some international sites as well. It may be necessary for students to travel to sites during at least a portion of the last year, depending on the availability of clinical rotations in their location.

Combined Degree Programs

Many schools today offer combined degree programs such as the PharmD/PhD, PharmD/MBA, PharmD/JD, PharmD/MPH, and even a PharmD/MS in Regulatory Science. Students interested in pursuing a combined degree program must be accepted by both programs and meet the respective admission requirements for each program at the same institution. Applying to a combined degree program will not increase your chances of getting into pharmacy school. Rather, these programs are especially designed to provide highly motivated students with a unique opportunity to specialize their course of study at a substantial savings in time and cost. If you are interested in these programs, you'll need to do some extra research—you want to make sure both components of the dual degree are ideal for you. A school may have a pharmacy program you love, but the other half of the degree's program may leave you cold. The goal is to strike a balance that works best for you.

PharmD/PhD

If you have a strong interest in pursuing a research career, then consider applying for the PharmD/PhD program. This combined degree program is administered jointly by the Graduate School and the School of Pharmacy at a particular university. The program integrates the professional pharmacy school curriculum with the graduate curricula in the sciences (pharmacology; pharmaceutical economics and policy; pharmaceutical sciences; experimental pharmacotherapy) to develop an accelerated course of study leading to both the PharmD and PhD degrees obtained at a substantial saving of time. Students in the program will be involved in research and training activities while completing the PharmD degree. This early exposure to research will enable them to subsequently complete their PhD degree requirements in a shorter period of time than completing the degrees separately.

This dual degree program is designed for highly motivated and qualified students who are seeking to combine clinical and basic sciences to train for translating basic science research into clinical applications. The purpose of the program is to prepare "clinical scientists" for careers in academia, government, or industrial settings. PharmD/PhD degree holders may work as professors at a university or researchers at a government agency or pharmaceutical company, among many other options.

PharmD/MBA

This combined degree program was developed in response to the growing demand for pharmacists to be knowledgeable in both pharmacy and business administration. As healthcare delivery becomes more complex and more concerned with cost-effectiveness, the knowledge gained by students in the areas of accounting, finance, decision making, personnel, strategic planning, and related areas becomes necessary for daily management operations. Enrollment in this program permits the completion of all pharmacy and business school requirements in a total of five years, one year less than would be required if a student were to complete each degree separately. Graduates of the PharmD/MBA program are in high demand for hospital pharmacy operations, management positions in government agencies, and corporate management in the pharmaceutical industry.

PharmD/JD

There is a growing need for health professionals with legal backgrounds and this combined degree program provides the opportunity to combine the expertise from both disciplines. Students can develop and combine various areas of expertise within both disciplines, such as product liability, intellectual property, and patent and professional responsibility law or geriatric and/or pediatric pharmacy with medical malpractice. Graduates from this program pursue careers in health-related law with the pharmaceutical industry (drug development), patent law, or private practice.

PharmD/MPH

If you have a strong interest in public health, you may consider pursuing the combined PharmD/MPH offered jointly by the pharmacy school and the school of public health. Candidates acquire the skills, knowledge, and awareness that define the public health perspective on healthcare. Graduates of this program are involved in public health programs and policy at the local, state, national, or international level. They may also prepare for academic careers, using their knowledge of epidemiology to conduct research in the clinical or public health sector or to implement community-based health programs.

PUBLIC VERSUS PRIVATE SCHOOLS: PREFERENCE FOR IN-STATE RESIDENTS

Some U.S. public pharmacy institutions give preference to in-state (resident) students. For this reason, you should take a close look at schools located in your home state when considering which schools you will apply to. Out-of-state (non-resident) and international applicants may compete for a limited number of positions or may be ineligible for admission, depending on institutional and state policies. Some private pharmacy institutions may offer a greater number of admissions positions to out-of-state and foreign applicants as compared to state-supported, public institutions. Be sure to check with your institutions of interest as to whether they have preference for in-state residents. Refer to the Resource section of this book for a listing of the private versus public pharmacy institutions as well as those that participate in the PharmCAS.

In conclusion, there are multiple factors that will play into finding the best pharmacy school for you. We strongly encourage you to review the tables in the Resource section of this book and spend time researching the programs available. The next chapter will tell you more about how to get to know the finer details about the list of schools you finally decide on.

CHAPTER 6

Researching Pharmacy Schools

Although it may be tempting to apply to schools without having researched them, succumbing to this temptation may get you into trouble later in the process. Pharmacy school admissions committees are most interested in an applicant whose decision to apply to their school is clearly an informed one. You should demonstrate enough specific interest in the school that the committee believes you would accept its offer over one from another school.

Therefore, one of the most important things you need to do—before even thinking about which schools to apply to—is the proper research so you can collect the necessary information you need about each school. The more you know about each school, the more comfortable and easier it will be for you when it comes time to choosing the right program for your pharmacy education. Pharmacy school admissions committees are interested in knowing that your decision to apply to their program is based on your knowledge of what they have to offer and how good a fit you are for their school. The decision you make needs to be an informed one. In other words, you need to make a strong argument for how you and your school of choice are a good match. The information you gather about each school will help you in answering some of the short essays on the supplemental application to the Pharmacy College Application Service (PharmCAS) as to why you are applying to or would be interested in attending that particular school. Additionally, you may be asked these same questions during your interview session. The more information you have, the better prepared you will be to lay out the specifics and the reasons as to why you're attracted to that school.

RESOURCES

There are numerous ways to research pharmacy schools and find out everything you need to know about their programs. Some resources include the Pharmacy School Admission Requirements (PSAR; as described in chapter 3) and the American Association of Colleges of Pharmacy (AACP) or pharmacy school websites as well as other online sources. Pharmacy school websites provide a glimpse of their program to you online. While some schools' websites may be easy to navigate, others may not be, or the information they provide may not be up-to-date. For complete information, it is always best to request the official school catalog. Most schools will usually hold on-campus tours or informational sessions for prospective students throughout the year. Attending one of these events is very useful because you will have the opportunity to meet with individuals in the admissions office, ask questions about their program and about financial aid, and even talk to current students about their experiences and find out the pros and cons of the school. More importantly, you will have a tour of the campus and get a feel of what it's like to actually be there if the school environment is a critical component of your decision-making process.

Inside Scoop Ask current pharmacy students about the schools they attend and how they got in. Not only will you get information on what worked for them in the application process, but you'll also get a sense of whether a particular school is right for you.

Talking to an alumnus of the school is another great way to find out more information about the institution. Joining the prepharmacy student association (if your undergraduate college has one) will also allow you to network and meet other potential applicants who may be researching pharmacy schools, and then you can pool your resources.

WEBSITES

Perusing pharmacy school websites can give you great insight into the specifics of a school. You should carefully read the online information for each school to which you're applying. The admissions committee will expect you to have read and familiarized yourself with the school's website before you complete the secondary application—and certainly before you show up for the interview. In addition, many pharmacy school websites have added personalized features that allow you to track the status of your application online.

Reading the Website

Keep in mind that a school's website is a marketing tool as well as a repository of information. Schools are interested in attracting the best students they can, so they put their best foot forward. (Undergraduate schools do the same thing, of course; take a look at the current brochure your undergraduate institution puts out and compare it with your personal experience.) Take the photos with a grain of salt. Although they can provide some valuable information, a good photographer can make any set of buildings look like a country club.

Many websites also profile some of the school's students. While the students profiled may be outstanding in some way or another, they are not necessarily representative of the average student at the school. So don't assume that you won't be a competitive applicant just because you didn't spend two years deep in the heart of Brazil learning about the medicinal properties of rare plants as the student pictured on the website did.

In addition to the admissions-related sections on the websites, you should look around on pages designed for current PharmD students. On those pages you will receive more inside information regarding the curriculum, social activities, and other issues or opportunities that the admissions office chose not to discuss on their website.

Glossy photos and student profiles notwithstanding, the website does contain a lot of information that is not only necessary to know for interviews, but will also help you compare that school to others you are interested in.

WHAT'S THE IMPORTANT INFORMATION?

The information you want to collect as you do your research includes any of the following areas discussed in the next sections.

Curriculum

Find out how the four-year program is structured (didactic versus experiential), what the coursework involves, and when the experiential component (e.g., externships, clinical rotations) takes effect. Some pharmacy schools offer a three-year, full-time, year-round program leading to the PharmD degree or even combined-degree programs such as the PharmD/PhD, PharmD/MBA, PharmD/JD, and PharmD/MPH.

Application Requirements

Identify the specific prerequisite coursework, necessity of the Pharmacy College Admission Test (PCAT), application deadlines, processing fees, and whether the school participates in the PharmCAS.

Selection Criteria

Certain schools may provide statistics on the enrollment of the students with regards to mean GPA, major, demographics, and whether preference is given to bachelor degree holders or in-state residential status. You can also find a good deal of this information in the Resources section of this book.

Financial Aid

Find out eligibility status, when and how to apply for assistance, and the availability of loans, grants, scholarships, and fellowship opportunities. (See Part Four for detailed information on how to tackle the financial aid process.)

Rankings

U.S. News & World Report provides rankings of pharmacy schools based on the results of peer assessment surveys sent to deans, other administrators, and/or faculty at accredited degree programs. In the fall of 2007, surveys were conducted for the 2008 rankings of PharmD programs accredited by the Accreditation Council for Pharmacy Education (ACPE) with a response rate of 56 percent. Thus, you need to be cautious when reading reports of school rankings. It is more important that you evaluate a school based upon factors that are important to you (see chapter 5 for more detail on ways to select a pharmacy program) rather than strictly on these rankings. Factors that may influence your decision to apply to a particular institution include program content, geographic location, faculty-to-student ratio, experiential training opportunities, student demographics, and cost.

Pharmacist Licensure Passing Rate

Find out what the passing rate is for graduates of the program when they take their pharmacist licensure exam, the North American Pharmacist Licensure Examination (NAPLEX).

Post-PharmD Activity

Find out what pharmacy practice areas the graduates end up going into (e.g., hospital versus community pharmacy, academia, research, managed care, etc.) and the percentage of those entering a residency or fellowship.

PART THREE

Applying to Pharmacy School—Navigating the Application Process

CHAPTER 7

Admissions Criteria

You should plan on applying to pharmacy school one year in advance of entering a program. For example, if you are currently enrolled in a four-year undergraduate college and plan on completing your bachelor's degree before entering pharmacy school, then you will need to complete the application process generally after you finish your third year of college. Keep in mind that each pharmacy school has its own admissions process with regards to requirements and application deadlines. It is always best to contact each school for the most up-to-date information.

In addition to completing the prepharmacy requirements, most pharmacy admissions committees will be evaluating potential applicants based on the following criteria:

ACADEMIC ABILITY

Admissions committees want to make sure that you will be able to handle the rigorous pharmacy curriculum you will face in their PharmD program. They will assess your academic potential by evaluating both your overall cumulative grade point average (GPA) (which includes all college coursework) and your prepharmacy GPA (which includes the prerequisite courses). As noted earlier, even an upward trend in grade performance will be viewed favorably, especially if you are trying to demonstrate an improvement in your GPA. Nonetheless, always try to maintain your GPA as high as possible.

How an admissions committee views your GPA, however, may be biased by where you went to undergraduate school, the courses you took, if there is evidence of grade inflation, and if there are any other mitigating circumstances in your application package.

Difficulty of Classes

It is well known in some competitive top-tier schools that a grade of C in organic chemistry is actually a very impressive grade. Thus, if you are applying to pharmacy schools near your undergraduate alma mater, your admissions officer may be very familiar with the particular professors and/or courses. They can look at a student's class grades and interpret how much harder it was to achieve the B in Physics as compared to the A in Anthropology.

Grade Inflation

The committee also considers grade inflation, which is prevalent at many schools (especially courses offered at community colleges). Committee members usually know which institutions tend to inflate and which don't, and they take that into account when evaluating your GPA.

Trends

Some pharmacy schools consider a positive trend in your GPA over time. If you got off to a slow start but have improved significantly in more recent semesters, this may work to your advantage. However, if your grades have gone down over time, this may be a problem.

Mitigating Circumstances

If you had an illness or family crisis that resulted in one semester or one year of weaker scores, be sure to address this up front in your personal statement. Furthermore, if you had a break in your education due to some unusual circumstance, again address this up front in your application. It is better to be honest and forthright than to have the committee guess about your career progression.

PHARMACY EXPERIENCE/KNOWLEDGE OF THE PHARMACY PROFESSION

Admissions committees want to know that you are familiar with the field of pharmacy. While they recognize that it is impossible for you to gain experience as a pharmacist, you can most certainly demonstrate that you have knowledge of and have gained some exposure to the profession. Thus, you are encouraged to shadow or observe a pharmacist, volunteer or work in a pharmacy-related or healthcare setting, or even conduct an interview with a pharmacist. The more you know about the profession, the better prepared you will be during your application process—from writing your personal statement to attending your interview. This is one of the most important criteria because it will help the committee determine your understanding of the profession.

LEADERSHIP SKILLS

Involvement in extracurricular activities will enable you to gain leadership skills. This will show the admissions committee that you have the potential to become a future leader in the field. Leadership is also a critical management skill that is utilized in the daily functions of a pharmacist, especially in running an effective pharmacy operation and even in managing staff.

EFFECTIVE COMMUNICATION

Having effective communication skills is very important to becoming a successful pharmacist—pharmacy is above anything else a people-oriented occupation. You will constantly be interacting with patients, physicians, nurses, and other members of the healthcare team. As such, you will need to be able to articulate to them your knowledge of drug information and drug therapy. Your oral and written communication skills are usually evaluated during the pharmacy interview, and some schools will even include a writing component to the interview process where you will be required to submit a writing sample. Further detail about the interview portion of admissions can be found in chapter 11.

COMMUNITY SERVICE

Your community service experience will show your interest in helping people and your commitment to giving back to your community. It is important to not only demonstrate your ability to work well with others, but also your willingness to learn from others. Both traits are hallmarks of the pharmacy profession.

THE NONTRADITIONAL STUDENT

By nontraditional students we mean those that come to pharmacy later in life. Admissions committees in general do not consider your age in the evaluation of your application—many individuals apply and are accepted to pharmacy school later on in their career. While this may not be the norm, these individuals do very well in the program and often are leaders in the profession following graduation. Reasons for delaying a pharmacy career vary: some may have taken time to raise a family; some might have served in the military immediately out of high school; and even some might have worked in the industry in some capacity after receiving a doctorate in pharmacy.

If you are applying as a nontraditional student, be up front in your personal statement about why those experiences have matured you and will make you a better pharmacy student and ultimately a better pharmacist. In addition, be sure to check with the coursework requirements of the institution to which you're applying—many schools require that your science and math college coursework be less than 5–10 years old, depending on the institutional policy. If your prerequisite courses were taken more than five years prior, check with the pharmacy admissions office directly to determine if you must retake these classes in order to be eligible for admission.

YOUR TOTAL PACKAGE

Admission to a pharmacy school can be competitive, but exact levels vary from year to year depending on the size and strength of the applicant pool. Admissions committees base their decision on an evaluation of all components of the application process: grades, experience, letters of recommendations, essays, personal statement, and interview. Although your GPA is an important factor, it is not the sole reason for acceptance to a pharmacy program. Admissions committees often look for well-rounded candidates, and typically select applicants with diverse backgrounds and experiences. Do not be afraid to highlight any unique talent, skill, attribute, or experience that you may have and explain how it has helped to develop you into the person you are. Also, remember to explain any personal extenuating circumstances that may have affected your academic achievement (e.g., working full-time while in school, family responsibilities, etc.). Don't try to hide something that has legitimately held you back from being the best you can be!

In addition to the above criteria, one very important aspect that the committee wants to assess is your motivation for pursuing a career in pharmacy. Thus, remember to communicate clearly both in your personal statement and during your interview your desire to pursue this profession.

CHAPTER 8

Completing the Application

The pharmacy school application is your single best opportunity to convince a group of strangers that you would be an asset both to its school and to the profession. It's your opportunity to show yourself as something more than grades and scores. Granted, every person who applies will have strengths and weaknesses, but it's how you present your strengths and weaknesses that counts.

So what's the best way to present yourself on the application? We all know that some people are natural-born sellers in person, but the majority of the admissions process is written, not oral. The key here is not natural talent but rather organization—carefully planning a coherent presentation from beginning to end and paying attention to every detail in between.

When you have the list of pharmacy schools that have made your cut, you will next need to determine the application procedures set forth by *each* school you're interested in applying to. Preparation is key in thoroughly completing your application. Before you begin filling out your application, find out what information you will need to collect for all sections of the application.

WHAT IS PHARMCAS?

The first fact you want to check is whether a school participates in the **Pharmacy College Application Service** (PharmCAS). PharmCAS is a centralized application service for colleges and schools of pharmacy provided by the American Association of Colleges of Pharmacy (AACP). Approximately three-fourths of all pharmacy programs in the United States participate in this service. (For a list of all pharmacy schools in the United States and whether they use PharmCAS, refer to the Resources section at the end of the book.) PharmCAS allows you to submit just one application, no matter how many schools you apply to. It is a web-based application where you can fill out the required forms on the PharmCAS website at www.pharmcas.org, and then submit them electronically. After submission of all required documentation, PharmCAS will assemble your application file, verify the accuracy of the information, calculate standardized grade point averages (GPAs), and electronically forward your application file to your designated pharmacy schools. Remember, this only works for schools that participate in this service. This service is designed specifically for first-year professional pharmacy degree applicants only. (Note: If you are a high school student applying to a six-year pharmacy degree program, a bachelor of science pharmacy degree graduate, or currently a pharmacy student who wishes to transfer to another pharmacy degree program, you should contact the institutions directly for specific instructions.)

The PharmCAS website is also a useful and helpful resource to learn more about the admissions process and requirements for each school. This site provides detailed instructions for completing the PharmCAS portion of the application process. Familiarize yourself with the full instructions provided on the website.

PharmCAS accepts applications beginning each spring for admission to pharmacy school in the fall of the following calendar year. For instance, if you are hoping to enter pharmacy school in Fall 2012, then you will complete the online PharmCAS application sometime between Spring 2011 and Fall 2011. It is important that you check with individual schools for their specific application deadlines.

To begin an application, you must visit the PharmCAS website to set up an account. You do not need to complete the entire PharmCAS application in one session. Once you have created an account, you may return at anytime through the submission deadline to work on your application.

Checklist for Applicants Who Apply through PharmCAS

- Submit a complete web application.
- Arrange to send official transcripts to PharmCAS.
- Send letters of recommendation and test scores to PharmCAS (if required by your designated pharmacy school).
- Submit the correct PharmCAS application fee.
- Do all of the above by the application deadline.

In addition to the PharmCAS, some pharmacy schools may require that you submit additional application materials, such as the supplemental application and fees, directly to the school. While this information is made available on the PharmCAS website, it is always safe practice to contact each school for comprehensive application instructions and deadlines.

DEADLINES

As mentioned earlier, allow plenty of time to complete your online application before the deadline approaches. Participating PharmCAS schools encourage you to submit applications at least two weeks before their institutional deadline to ensure timely processing and to help avoid delays (from web congestion due to a high number of applicants and Internet traffic especially around the time of deadlines). Find out which schools offer a "rolling admissions" process or give special consideration to applicants who submit applications earlier in the admissions cycle. Submitting your materials early to these particular programs may improve your chances for admission.

NON-PHARMCAS SCHOOLS

About one-fourth of the U.S. pharmacy institutions do not participate in PharmCAS. These programs require that you apply directly to the schools by completing their individual applications. You will need to contact these schools for specific application instructions and to request application forms.

> **Follow Directions**
>
> Admissions officers are amazed at how many applicants simply refuse to follow directions. Don't think that you're an exception to any rule. If the application asks for X, give them X, not Y.

APPLICATION DOS AND DON'TS

1. *Triple-check your application for spelling errors.*

   You lose a certain amount of credibility if you write that you were a "Roads Scholar." Ask a family member or friend to read through your application as well.

2. *Check for accidental contradictions.*

   Make sure your application doesn't say that you worked in a hospital in 1995 when your financial aid forms say you were driving a cab that year.

3. *Prioritize all lists.*

   When you're asked to list your honors or awards, don't begin with fraternity social chairman and end with Phi Beta Kappa. Let the admissions committee know that you realize what's important—always list significant scholastic accomplishments first.

4. *Account for all of your time.*

   If you have been away from school for longer than a semester, did not enter college directly from high school, have been out of college for some time, or had other breaks in your education, be sure that your application shows what you were doing during that period. Don't leave gaps.

5. *Don't overdo listing extracurricular activities.*

   Don't list every activity you ever participated in. Select the most significant and, if necessary, explain them. Admissions officers are suspicious of people who list 25 time-consuming extracurriculars and yet still manage to attend college. Ask a close friend to help you select the most significant activities to list and discuss.

6. ***Don't mention high school activities or honors.***
   Unless there's something very unusual or spectacular about your high school background, don't mention it. Yes, this means not stating that you were senior class president. However, do list health-related work or volunteering.

7. ***Clear up any ambiguities.***
   On questions concerning employment, for instance, make sure to clarify whether you held a job during the school year or only over the summer. Many applications ask about this, and it may be an important point to the admissions officer.

Just the Facts, Ma'am

"Be careful not to overstate facts on your applications. I've looked at thousands of applications and can quickly see fluff."

—Robert, admissions officer

CHAPTER 9

Personal Statement

The personal statement portion of your application is an opportunity to present yourself to the admissions committee. This is the best time for you to tell others your story and to write out your personal and professional goals; your statement should be a reflection of your aptitude, maturity, focus, and compatibility with the profession of pharmacy. The personal statement also provides evidence of your writing skills. Because of all that it holds, the personal statement is a critical factor in the admissions process. Writing a unique, powerful statement can only be to your benefit.

IDEAS FOR GETTING STARTED

As a basic guideline, your statement should address why you have chosen pharmacy, how you know that this is the right choice for you, and what you have to offer the profession. If you have trouble getting started, remember first and foremost to just be yourself—this is the best way to showcase your unique and genuine side and passion for what you believe in.

Let the admissions committee get to know you by providing insight into your personality and your life goals and dreams. Describe what got you interested in this field. Explain your professional objectives after pharmacy school. You may want to discuss how any

---

Weave a Story

Use vignettes and anecdotes to add interest to your essay. Why did you decide to go into pharmacy? Was it an experience you had in school? Have you or family members had an experience with the pharmacy community that left a lasting impression? Be creative!

---

applied learning experiences you have had (e.g., work, volunteering, internship) have contributed to your professional objectives. This is also the time to demonstrate how your research and/or clinical experiences relate to your ultimate professional goals. You can justify how your academic choices reflect your interests and will prepare you for a career in pharmacy.

EXPLAINING SPECIAL CIRCUMSTANCES

You may also use the personal statement to explain or present any special circumstances. For example, you may want to consider writing about a semester with low grades, a switch in major, gaps in enrollment, or reasons you are applying as a nontraditional applicant. When you are writing about these special circumstances, remember to focus on your strength and resilience, addressing how you've learned from the situation or describing the experience you've gained. Admissions officers are interested in knowing how your unique experiences have shaped you and how you handle your challenges in life; therefore, you should discuss in detail how you've matured from the experiences you've encountered. Keep in mind that circumstances shouldn't be the main focus of your essay, but rather peripheral to the story.

FINE-TUNING YOUR STATEMENT

Whatever you decide to write about, you should structure your statement to include relevant (academic or work-related) experience that has contributed to your professional maturity. Mention awards and honors, leadership positions in school organizations, and writing or publishing experience. However, make sure that your statement is not just a restatement of your résumé. Essentially, your personal statement should provide the framework for the supplemental application essay questions. Give yourself plenty of time to write by starting early because any writing project requires you to go through several rounds of revisions. Other writing tips include being specific rather than vague by providing examples, being coherent and concise, and writing a positive statement revealing realistic and achievable goals. Try to link personal information to professional interests and/or goals.

When you have completed writing your statement, it is always wise to get a second opinion. Ask others to help review your statement. Choose someone who knows you well and will be honest. Find another person you know who writes well so that they can help edit your statement. Always remember to proofread what you write. Admissions committees are looking for you to display strong written communication skills; thus, high-quality writing is expected in the personal statement.

WRITING DRAFTS

Because the personal statement is such an important part of your application, it shouldn't be done overnight. A strong personal statement may take shape over the course of weeks or months and will require several different drafts. Write a draft and then let it sit for a few weeks. Time gives you valuable perspective on something you've written. If you leave it alone for a significant period of time, you may find (to your astonishment) that your first instincts were good ones; on the other hand, you may shudder at how you could ever have considered submitting something so horrific!

Allow at least a month or so to write your statement, and don't be afraid to overhaul it completely if you're not satisfied. Most important, get several different perspectives. Have close friends or relatives read it to see if it really captures what you want to convey, asking them about their initial reaction as well as their feelings after studying it more carefully. Once you've achieved a draft that you feel comfortable with, have a few people who barely know you read it. Because they haven't heard the story before and don't know the characters, they're often able to tell you when something is missing or confusing.

The bottom line is to let a reasonable number of people read the essay and make suggestions. To avoid being overly influenced by an individual reader, try to read all of the comments at once. If certain criticisms are consistently made, then they're probably legitimate. But don't be carried away by every suggestion every reader makes. Stick to your basic instincts—after all, this is your personal statement.

> ### Proofread!
> Proofreading is of critical importance. Don't be afraid to enlist the aid of others. If possible, let an English teacher review the essay solely for spelling and grammar mistakes. Nothing catches an admissions officer's eye more quickly than a misspelled word.

THE FIVE MOST COMMON MISTAKES

We asked an admissions officer for the five most common mistakes students make in writing their personal statements. Here's what she told us:

1. Underestimating the Importance of the Essay

It appears to be a common misperception that a stellar academic record will overcome other deficiencies in a student's application, including a poorly written personal statement. This is often glaringly evident when a student writes a few hastily constructed paragraphs, leaving most of the allotted page blank. In other less obvious examples, students simply don't allot enough time to polish the essay.

2. Using Excessive Detail–the "Overwhelm and Conquer" Approach

This common misperception—that more is better—results in an essay that generates groans from the unfortunate reader on the admissions committee. Unfortunately, it is such an unpleasant experience for the reader to wade through this essay that the entire application often goes to the bottom of the pile.

3. Failing to Make the Essay Personal

Another common mistake is to use the essay to recite a list of activities and accomplishments, without really addressing the question, "Why pharmacy?" When students fail to convey what they learned from their experiences, they fail to communicate to an admissions committee how they see themselves as an asset to the pharmacy profession. Ask your mother and your best friend to review your personal statement to make sure they can hear your "voice" in it.

4. Embellishing the Essay

Students often avoid the personal approach entirely by writing an overly creative or philosophical treatise, hoping to impress the committee with their unique approach. While this approach may be interesting reading, it does not leave the reader with a compelling reason to recommend the student for an interview. There is a place for creativity in the essay, but overall, the personal statement should not deviate from the standard essay format.

5. Failing to Proofread the Essay

Attention to detail often eludes the pharmacy school applicant. The failure to proofread can be a devastating mistake, because nothing destroys the credibility of an application faster than misspelled words and faulty grammar. Admissions committees place a high value on strong communication skills—both written and verbal—and expect high-quality writing in the personal statement.

THE SUPPLEMENTAL APPLICATION TO THE PHARMCAS

Some pharmacy admissions programs that participate in the PharmCAS may require you to submit a supplemental application where you are asked to answer additional essay questions regarding your interest in the pharmacy profession. Check with each individual institution on its requirements for submitting this supplemental application.

The supplemental application is designed to provide admissions committee members another opportunity to learn more about you as a person—what are the unique experiences, interests, and skills you possess that separate you from the rest of the applicant pool. For example, you may be asked to expand upon information you listed in the PharmCAS application with regards to extracurricular, leadership, volunteer, and community activities, and/or work experience. You may be asked to provide evidence of your leadership ability by elaborating on the above-listed experience and to discuss your level of involvement and the skills, knowledge, and insight you have gained from this endeavor. Admissions officers are interested in determining the depth of your commitment and learning how you weigh your experiences in terms of value. Another question you may be asked is to use examples from your own life to address some of the implications of the growing cultural diversity that exists in our society and determine the impact this will have on pharmacy practice. You may also be asked to discuss how you will contribute to the diversity that exists in the school's PharmD program.

We understand that these may be difficult questions, but they are thought-provoking questions aimed at testing your intellectual ability and your awareness of a profession that is constantly changing. Don't take these questions lightly. Take the time to outline how you are going to approach your response. Again, allow yourself plenty of time to answer all essays to your satisfaction. Do not wait until the approaching deadline to finish the supplemental portion of your application.

A subsection of the supplemental application is reserved for applicants reapplying to a PharmD program. If you are reapplying, you would use this space to describe how you have changed and strengthened your application from the previous application cycle. You will want to include any relevant academic, work, volunteer, personal, or pharmacy experience that you have acquired over the past year to increase the competitiveness of your application this year. Above all, be sure to address each and every way you have prepared to be a better candidate this year.

CHAPTER 10

Letters of Recommendation

Letters of recommendation (also known as letters of evaluation) are typically required and submitted as part of the application process. The most important point you should take from this chapter is to start thinking about soliciting your letters early on in the process. It may take a good amount of time for your letter writers, who are busy professionals, to complete them. Many pharmacy programs require from one to three letters of recommendation as part of the pharmacy admissions process. Schools may request that you submit letters from particular evaluators, such as a pharmacist, professor, or academic advisor. You may also request letters from supervisors from work and volunteer experiences, and from guidance counselors who know your work and future plans.

GENERAL GUIDELINES

Look for people who you are positive can write you good letters of recommendation. Be sure to choose those individuals who know you and your work well and with whom you have a close relationship, such as a shared interest in academic and/or professional matters. Make sure whomever you choose can speak to your maturity, dependability, dedication, compassion, communication skills, leadership, and any hands-on experience in the field. When you approach

---

The Best of the Best

"Almost all letters of recommendations will be positive...but as an admissions committee we are looking for superlatives:

"This is one of the best students I've had...."

"Extremely bright and hardworking...."

"A must for your program...."

"A true leader...."

—James, pharmacy school admissions officer

someone to write a letter of recommendation, don't hesitate to ask whether she can write you a strong letter of support. If you sense that she hesitates in any way ("I'm very busy now"; "I'm going to be out of town"), then look elsewhere. This may be her way of telling you that she can't or won't write a strong letter for you. Although this may be embarrassing, it will hurt you a lot more in the long run to have someone's late recommendation force you to withdraw your application, or worse yet, to have a lukewarm letter of recommendation submitted.

> ### Stay Away from Strangers
> Beware of the impersonal recommendation. Be sure to ask a potential recommender if he or she can write a strong letter. If not, move on.

If you have been out of school for several years, be sure to select recommenders (e.g., a supervisor from work or a volunteer coordinator) who are able to write about your intellectual ability, communication skills, and personal qualities in detail. If you have returned to school to fulfill prerequisites, you may also decide to ask your current instructors to speak to your abilities.

HOW TO SOLICIT LETTERS

Having to approach a professor to ask for a letter of recommendation can be a daunting experience. This is particularly true if you are planning to approach a professor whose class you attended years ago, or one in which you were one of 300 students. The concern, and it is a very real concern, is that letters solicited under these circumstances will be no more than glorified form letters and will be written with very little insight.

Your job, therefore, is to put yourself in a position in which your professors get to know you. Notice that we didn't tell you to "put yourself in a position in which you get to know your professors." That misses the point. You're not writing your professor a letter of recommendation; he or she is writing one for you. So how do you help your professor get to know you? Step one: Start early.

While you're completing your prepharmacy requirements, visit your professor during office hours if you have any questions regarding course material. Students will often seek out their teaching assistant's for assistance, but seldom their professors. Chances are that if you go to see your professor during office hours, you will be one of only a handful of students present. Consider getting a cup of coffee with your professor.

Many undergraduate institutions sponsor something called "Take Your Professor to Lunch" to encourage faculty and students to intermingle. What a deal: Not only do you get a free lunch, but you also get to know your professors outside of the classroom. And if you do well in a particular class or have an especially positive experience, apply to become a teaching assistant the following year or volunteer to work in that professor's lab. The possibilities are limitless; you just need to put forth a little effort to get the relationship started.

Assuming the individuals you ask express pleasure and honor at being requested to write a letter on your behalf, be prepared to give them a copy of your résumé to provide a complete picture of your background and interests. If you have a strong academic record, you may want to include a copy of your transcript. Any articles or papers that you think may be helpful should also be offered. Finally, always provide recommenders with addressed and stamped envelopes to the school in question.

ETIQUETTE

Again, always give your letter writers plenty of time to write a strong and solid letter and to be sure that they submit them on time. Thus, it is important to solicit your letters as early as possible. Don't wait until the fall to ask for letters of recommendation. You don't want to be crushed in the fall rush, when zillions of students are scrambling and science professors are overwhelmed. Waiting until the last minute means that it's likely that the quality of the letters will suffer.

Provide recommenders with addressed and stamped envelopes to the schools to which they should be sent, unless the institution participates in the PharmCAS letter of recommendation service (where letters are submitted directly to PharmCAS). We will discuss the PharmCAS process in detail later in the chapter.

Keep track of the status of your letters. If they're late, call and check on their progress. But don't harass your recommenders; if you make a pest of yourself, it could negatively impact what they will end up writing about you. Once you've confirmed that your letters have been sent, it's nice to send thank-you notes to the writers. Personal visits are in order after you've been accepted.

WHAT MAKES A GREAT RECOMMENDATION?

Keep in mind the purpose of recommendation letters: They serve as outside endorsements of your pharmacy school candidacy. The more personal the letter, the better off you are. Schools fully expect these letters to be glowing endorsements. Anything less is a red flag. Admissions committees are looking for applicants who have demonstrated intelligence, maturity, integrity, and a dedication to the idea of service to society—all the things that you'd look for in a pharmacist. To this end, a glowing letter of recommendation generally begins by detailing the circumstances under which the letter writer has come to know the applicant. This includes the length of time and the nature of the association. It then evaluates the candidate on the nature and depth of scholarly and/or extracurricular activities undertaken, the candidate's academic record and performance on PCATs, the personal and emotional characteristics of the candidate, and finally, the letter writer's overall assessment as to the candidate's suitability for the pharmacy profession. The admissions committee may consider detrimental a letter of recommendation that focuses solely on the academic qualifications of the applicant and gives little or no attention to the candidate's nonacademic strengths and characteristics.

THE PHARMCAS LETTERS OF REFERENCE SERVICE

Many colleges and schools participate in the PharmCAS online letters of reference service. To apply to institutions that accept letters via the PharmCAS, you should either direct your evaluators to the site where they can use the electronic letters of reference (eLORs) form or can download a copy of the form available on the PharmCAS. You can enter up to four evaluator names on your PharmCAS application. Before you begin, be sure to review the PharmCAS School Reference Table to learn the number of letters required and types of acceptable evaluators for each institution. Keep in mind, however, this only pertains to those institutions that participate in the service. You cannot rely on the PharmCAS site to determine if you have met the reference requirements for a particular pharmacy school. Also, be advised that PharmCAS will not forward letters to pharmacy schools that do not accept them—a few pharmacy institutions prefer that applicants send letters directly to the schools. Make sure to review the admission requirements of each individual school for specific instructions and deadlines. PharmCAS will forward up to three references to all of your designated pharmacy schools, regardless of the school's preference.

If your school of choice accepts them, strongly encourage your evaluators to send eLORs to PharmCAS. Paper references take longer to duplicate and send to your designated pharmacy schools. If your evaluator chooses to use the paper reference, provide him with the PharmCAS Evaluation Form and have him attach it to the reference letter. Pharmacy schools may not accept paper references unless a completed form and letter are attached. Paper references must be mailed to PharmCAS in a sealed envelope (with the letter of reference and PharmCAS reference form together inside) on the evaluator's signed official institutional or business stationery. PharmCAS will not accept paper references mailed by applicants. PharmCAS then will provide a copy of your paper reference to each of your designated pharmacy schools.

Be sure to arrange for PharmCAS to receive all of your letters by the earliest application deadline date set by your designated pharmacy schools. Some pharmacy schools will not consider applicants who submit late materials. PharmCAS does NOT enforce reference deadlines and will forward the references to your designated schools even if they arrive late. Be sure to visit the PharmCAS website at www.pharmcas.org for detailed information on this service.

CONFIDENTIAL OR NONCONFIDENTIAL LETTERS

Prior to requesting a reference from an evaluator, you are required to indicate whether you wish to waive your rights to have full access to your letters of recommendations. PharmCAS will release your decision to waive or not to waive access to your evaluator and your designated pharmacy schools. Some admissions committees interpret references as more honest and candid if you waive your right to see the letters. If you do not waive your rights, you may be asked to explain the reason for your choice during the interview process.

> **Do the Waive**
>
> Conventional wisdom dictates that you should waive your option to review your recommendations. Pharmacy schools prefer that you not have any hand in what is written about you in these letters.

Again, we cannot emphasize enough that you should not wait until the fall to ask for your letters of recommendation because this is the period when other pharmacy candidates are rushing to solicit their letters as well. Allow your evaluators plenty of time to prepare and get your letter in on time. Keep track of the status of your letters. It is okay to give gentle reminders to your evaluators of approaching deadlines, but do not constantly harass them. Once you've confirmed that your letters have been sent, it is a nice gesture to send thank-you notes to your letter writers. Definitely keep them informed of your final decision as they would appreciate knowing that their letter helped you get into the school of your choice.

CHAPTER 11

The Interview

Many pharmacy schools will invite competitive applicants to visit their campus for an interview. The admissions committee uses the interview process to make determinations on admissions. The purpose of an in-person interview is to assess your oral communication skills, writing skills, leadership ability, problem-solving and critical thinking skills, and motivation or potential to be a pharmacist. Whereas the first round in the admissions process—reviewing your numbers—may seem impersonal, the interview introduces an element of humanity. Here is where you can let your personality and charm really shine through.

The interview experience is multidimensional. Obviously, it is a time for the admissions committee to check you out, which means it is also a time for you to "show your stuff." However, you should also approach the interview day as a chance to determine whether you would want to attend that particular pharmacy school, assuming you have multiple acceptances.

THE ORAL PORTION OF THE INTERVIEW

Most interviews consist of two parts: an oral interview and a writing test. Interview format varies by institution—pharmacy colleges may require you to speak with a single faculty member, a student, a pharmacist, or a panel of interviewers. The oral interview also may be a two-person team, such as a faculty member and an advanced-standing student pharmacist. Although a major focus of the interview is to assess

---

Know Your Stuff

"During my interview of potential students, I'm looking for someone who has a clear reason for wanting to attend pharmacy school and who has done their homework on our university and the profession as a whole."

—Ken, pharmacy school admissions counselor

---

your communication skills, the interviewers also will be interested in your knowledge of pharmacy and your motivation to enter the profession. Admissions committees expect you to have researched the pharmacy profession and know some of the pivotal issues pharmacists currently face. You can research the field by browsing websites of pharmacy organizations such as the American Pharmacists Association (*www.pharmacist.com*), or by reading the publication *Pharmacy Times (www.pharmacytimes.com)*. You also should read the health section of the daily newspaper and pay attention to articles on big topics in pharmacy today. Do a keyword search on "pharmacy" if you are accessing these publications online. Because you may be asked to provide your viewpoint on the drug use process or review the state of pharmacy care today, you should be familiar with the scope of practice, the outcomes of medication therapy, and how technology integration influences the practice of pharmacy. Be sure to articulate your ideas clearly and present examples whenever possible to best illustrate what you mean.

Bone Up

It's a good idea to keep a copy of your written application with the school's catalog so you can review them both the night before your interview. Don't be caught off guard by questions on information you spoke about in your application.

Additionally, the admissions committee will want to know specifically why you are interested in pharmacy. Here is your opportunity to describe your pharmacy-related experiences and/or extracurricular activities. You'll want to talk about how they have shaped you professionally and academically up to this point, and also about how they will prepare you for a career in the pharmacy field. You should be prepared to discuss why you have chosen to pursue a career in the pharmacy profession and how you perceive the role of the pharmacist in healthcare. This is even more of a reason to have field experience through jobs or internships before you apply to pharmacy school—if you have researched or gained direct exposure to the profession, then you will be better prepared to respond to the interview questions.

Be Prepared for Anything!

Some interviews are very relaxed (they want to get to know you), others are more high pressure (they want to see how you respond to rapid questions, difficult questions, and difficult situations). Some schools have their applicants interview in conference rooms, others take them to professors' offices (while this might result in more distractions, it can also present more of an opportunity to find a common interest).

Some interviews are open-file while others are closed-file. An **open-file** interview means that the interviewer has already reviewed your application and will often begin the interview by referring to something you've included in your application. Therefore, remember to review your application materials before going into this type of interview. In a **closed-file** interview (sometimes referred to as a "blind" interview), the interviewer has never seen your application folder and may begin with a very open-ended question (such as "Tell me a little about yourself") as an icebreaker to get you warmed up. Before this type of interview, think about how you'll launch into talking about yourself if the interviewer has no prior information about you.

Group Interviews

Some schools only conduct one-on-one interviews (or two-on-one interviews), while others conduct group interviews with several candidates at once to see how you compare to others.

In a group interview, you might have three interviewers and three interviewees in a room. After an introduction and a generic, "loosen up" question, each of the interviewers gets to ask questions to each interviewee. Given time constraints, there is usually just time for one question apiece from each of the interviewers, which may not be the same for each interviewee. (For example, "John, tell me more about how your internship experience affected your rela-

> **Tips for Groupies**
> Etiquette tips for group interviews:
> - Don't hog the airtime.
> - Refer to others' answers if you get the same question after them.
> - Try not to take yourself too seriously.

tionship to pharmacy." "Mabel, how do you see changes in healthcare affecting how the pharmacy field operates?") Group interviews are designed for a school to gauge how well you "play with others," and whether you can share airtime, while being charming and eloquent, too.

Common Questions and Scenarios Presented During the Oral Interview

- Why do you want to be a pharmacist?
- Where do you see yourself in 10–15 years?
- Clearly describe your involvement in any community programs or activities outside the academic classroom, and the role your contributions played in the success of the activity, program, or organization.
- Give a brief history of your work experience and describe your duties and responsibilities.
- Explain the factors that have influenced your decision to pursue a career in pharmacy.
- Indicate any additional information you feel will be helpful in our appraisal of your application.
- Tell us a little bit about yourself other than what is stated in these essays.
- Why pharmacy?
- Why this school versus one of the other schools of pharmacy?
- Where do you see yourself in the future?
- What different fields in pharmacy are you interested in?
- What class, other than the pharmacy prerequisites, have you taken that has had an impact on your life?
- What would you do if you didn't get in this year?
- What do you do to relieve stress?
- *A common question involves a scenario in which a fellow student had not been able to finish an assignment:* Would you allow a fellow student to cheat or copy your assignment?
- *A reality question:* How many people are there in the world and how many are in the United States?
- What do you do for fun?
- What volunteer experiences have you been involved in?
- What leadership opportunities have you been involved with?
- What aspects of your life do you excel in?
- What has been your favorite class during college?
- What sets you apart from all the other applicants who have applied?

- *A clinical question:* A customer comes into a drug store right before closing on the weekend with no refills on their blood pressure and pain medicine. How would you handle the situation?
- Do you work well in groups?
- What is your approach to solving conflicts within a group?

Above all, be prepared—research each school you will interview at and know something about what makes each program stand apart from the others. Read the websites and any documents sent to you via mail. Be prepared to answer why you want to go to a particular school and why it should accept you. In other words, how can you contribute to its program? Definitely have a solid knowledge about the pharmacy profession. Try to come across confident, but don't appear to be arrogant. It is important to be courteous, and not appear confrontational. If challenged, be prepared to think on your feet—but don't get frustrated, irritated, or angry. Remain calm, don't get stressed out, and don't forget to smile! Most importantly, never criticize anyone (e.g., an old professor, a previous student, a past school). Be positive! Often, at the end of an interview, you will be asked by the interviewer if you have any questions. We recommend that you be prepared to ask questions—this shows that you are engaged in the interview process and that you are interested in what the school can offer *you* as a pharmacy student.

THE WRITTEN PORTION OF THE INTERVIEW

Following the oral interview, you will be given a limited amount of time (30–45 minutes) to write an essay on one of several topics. These topics are usually not academic in nature, nor do they test your knowledge in specific subjects. They may be more general questions and not pharmacy related. You may be asked to discuss a particular idea using examples from literature, personal experience, or current events. As such, while it is impossible to prepare for what to expect as essay topics, you can absolutely prepare on how to respond to the essay by brushing up on your writing ability. In fact, this essay exercise is designed to help the admissions committee assess your writing skills and development of ideas, as well as your problem-solving and critical thinking abilities.

Approach this essay as you would any English composition, providing an introductory paragraph, a body with supporting details, and a conclusion to summarize your response. Remember to review the steps on writing an essay with logical organization and be clear and concise on your ideas, providing adequate details or examples. Some schools require that you write this essay longhand, while others provide a computer for you to type your essay. If there is space restriction, you should plan your essay accordingly to ensure it fits within the allotted space. Remember to write legibly, use proper grammar, and answer in complete sentences.

Sample Essay Questions During the Written Interview Process

- What animal best represents you and what characteristics does it possess that best describe you?
- Have any of your classes during your college career helped to shape your values, and if so, how?
- Why have you chosen to become a pharmacist and what qualities do you feel are needed to be considered an exceptional pharmacist?
- What is the meaning of having a fulfilling life? Provide three examples and compare and contrast their values.
- Childhood obesity is a rising concern in the United States. Should kids be allowed to dictate what they eat or should there be some sort of parental control? What are some issues that need to be addressed?
- Should all students be required to take a psychology class in college? Why or why not?
- If you have one day to change this world, what would you change and how would you do it?

HOW TO PREPARE

As we said before, don't even think about going into your interviews cold. You need to prepare well in advance. You'll need to think about not only what you may encounter once you're facing your interviewer, but also when you'll interview, how you'll get there, how you'll behave, and what you'll wear.

Your best resources when preparing for the interview will include your prepharmacy advisor, students currently attending the pharmacy schools to which you are applying, and the school's catalog.

Scheduling

Your interview invitations will probably arrive at approximately the same time. Remember, for schools with rolling admissions, the sooner you have your interview, the sooner you'll be considered for acceptance. Most schools usually have prescheduled interview days and provide you with that date on your invitation to the interview. In this situation, you would not be able to determine the schedule of your interview. However, if a school allows you to schedule your interview, then do so as early as possible. Many students will try to schedule interviews at less competitive schools earlier, to gain interview experience and overcome early jitters. However, don't postpone your other interviews too long because it will delay completion of your applications.

Financial reasons may compel you to try to schedule groups of interviews in particular geographic regions. For instance, you may want to set up a West Coast interview tour and visit several schools in the same area during one trip. If you get one interview in a far-flung region and haven't yet heard from another school in the same area, don't hesitate to give the second school a call. Politely ask, "I'll be in this region on such and such a date interviewing at So and So. If you are planning to interview me, would it be possible to schedule an appointment near that time so I can make only one plane trip?" Schools will usually ask to get back to you, go look at your file, and then tell you yes if they are planning to interview you. If they're already booked for that time, they may offer another time slot.

Travel and Accommodations

It is at this point that the whole application process can really begin to get expensive. You probably know that you can keep costs down by making airline reservations as far in advance as possible and staying over a Saturday night. But did you know that major airlines often offer discounts to applicants for interview travel? It might also be worth your while to check with discount travel agents. They frequently have discounted tickets for sale, even if you give only a few days' notice. One other air travel tip: Carry your luggage with you on the plane. The last thing you want on interview day is to have your luggage sent to the wrong place.

Always do research in advance to find out about parking or the best way to reach the school from the airport. Usually, your interview offer will include directions to the school and information on accommodations. Some pharmacy schools have programs that allow you to stay with a student for free. Although a complimentary room may be economically enticing, remember that it's important for you to be comfortable. If sleeping on the floor of a student's apartment is going to stress you out, you'd be better off staying at the nearest budget motel. On the other hand, if money is short and you can find a student with an extra bed, it may be a good opportunity to get an inside scoop on the school's personality. Also, just as the pharmacy student touring you around can give you great information and affect how you view the school, someone you stay with can have an impact on your admission. It therefore behooves you to treat your host with respect. Remember, you are a guest in his or her home. Don't be demanding, don't expect your host to act as a taxi service, don't hog all the hot water for your shower in the morning, and remember to clean up after yourself.

If at all possible, arrive the night before the interview to familiarize yourself with the area and the school. This way, you won't have to worry about travel delays the day of your interview, and you also will have the opportunity to unwind and get a good night's sleep.

What to Wear

Professional attire is recommended for the interview. You are discouraged from wearing jeans, shorts, t-shirts, tank tops, bare midriffs, tennis shoes, flip-flops, or other attire that is considered inappropriate in a business environment. For men, a dark suit and an attractive (but not too flashy) tie are usually safe. Facial hair should be groomed, and go easy on the cologne. For women, a suit or dress is fine, but be careful of the hem length (you don't want it to be too short). Also, go easy on the jewelry, makeup, and perfume. Make sure to check the local weather and select your attire accordingly.

Online Assistance

A website that most students find very useful in helping them prepare for their interview is the Student Doctor Network (SDN) Pharmacy School Interview Feedback. (Go to www.studentdoctor.net/interview-feedback/, then under the interview feedback categories, select pharmacy school.) You can select any pharmacy school and read about other people's interview experiences at that particular school. You can pick up helpful tips for the interview process at that institution, view sample interview questions, and learn what the students thought about the school and their overall interview experience.

Advice from the Inside

We asked an admissions committee member for some pointers on interview day. Here's what she told us:

- Be incredibly nice to the school admissions secretary. He or she can be your best ally or your worst enemy.
- It's fine to bring in bags if your flight leaves immediately after the interview.
- Most schools offer coffee when you first arrive. Be aware that caffeine can make you nervous.
- Don't try to outdo the competition by comparing stats or name-dropping while waiting in the "greeting" room.
- Don't be vocal about not wanting to go to that school, even casually. "This is my safety" can safely ensure you won't get an offer.
- Do your homework and be prepared to ask questions.

LAST-MINUTE TIPS ON PREPARING FOR YOUR INTERVIEW DAY

The interview counts toward a significant portion in evaluating your overall application. As such, you want to prepare adequately for this important day. The following are some last-minute tips:

- Remember to have a good night's rest the day before.
- Bring personal identification (e.g., driver's license), your letter of invitation from the college, and a writing utensil.
- Allow yourself plenty of time to get to the institution on the day of the interview. It is better to arrive early than be late.
- Make sure you eat a good meal before your meeting so that you have the energy to last through the day. It may be embarrassing if your stomach growls during your oral interview session.
- Introduce yourself and shake hands firmly (this tip is for both males and females).
- Maintain eye contact, especially when asked a question.
- Do not chew gum or have candy in your mouth.
- Don't fidget.

- Don't cross your arms.
- Don't touch any items on the interviewer's desk or on the conference table.
- Speak loud enough so that the interviewer can hear and slow enough that he or she can comprehend.
- Smile at appropriate times.
- Don't be flirtatious.
- Avoid being arrogant and dogmatic (instead, try to come across as confident).
- If the interviewer is challenging you, do not answer in kind. Think before speaking. Do not raise your voice. Speak slowly. Be cool and composed.
- If you don't know the answer to a question, don't be afraid to say that you don't know. Do not try to make something up because more than likely the interviewer will be able to see right through you.
- After the interview:
  - Shake hands and say good-bye.
  - Let them know you are very interested in attending the school.

Remember, get your applications completed as early as possible because many institutions offer interviews on a rolling basis. If you are currently in school, it makes it really difficult to focus on coursework when you are worrying about completing applications and later scheduling your interviews. In fact, you might want to set a goal that you'll have all PharmCAS materials turned in by mid-August and all supplemental applications turned in as soon as they are available online.

Most students agree that interviews get easier with practice. For this reason, some recommend that you schedule your top choice school last, after you've become a pro at the interviewing game. Finally, be sure to contact the pharmacy admissions office immediately if you are unable to attend the interview on time or as scheduled, or if you no longer wish to be considered for admission.

CHAPTER 12

Admissions Process—
An Inside Perspective

Admission to any PharmD program is highly competitive due to the great number of well-qualified applicants. Assuming many pharmacy students are seemingly qualified—with good grade point averages (GPAs), respectable Pharmacy College Admission Test (PCAT) scores, prerequisites in place, and maybe even work/volunteer experience—how do pharmacy schools make their cuts? What are the factors that really count the most? Many admissions committees go through an initial review of your completed application to determine who will be invited for an on-campus interview. In this chapter, we will take a look at what happens to your completed application once it arrives in the admissions office.

WEIGHING IN ON THE FACTORS

Let's examine all the components of an application to see how an admissions committee breaks it down to make its final decisions.

Grade Point Average

The admissions committee is looking for applicants who have demonstrated strong academic ability—particularly in the prerequisite coursework listed in chapter 3, but also throughout their entire academic career. How your GPA is viewed is based on where you went to school, the particular classes you took, whether your grades are inflated, and if there are any other mitigating circumstances you use to explain discrepancies on your transcript. The admissions committee pays careful attention to the quality, rigor, and special circumstances of the prepharmacy record presented by each applicant. Thus, the committee may view your GPA with regards to how tough your school really was to determine the actual value of your GPA in its eyes. Some schools recommend that you take your prepharmacy coursework in the most demanding curricular environment possible. The admissions committee not only considers the strength of your undergraduate institution but also if it has admitted other students from the same institution and how well these former students are currently performing at that school.

The difficulty of the classes you have taken will also be considered. If you are applying to schools near your undergraduate college, you can expect that the local admissions officers are often acquainted with the professors and degree of difficulty of the classes. They can look at individual class grades and interpret how much harder you had to work for the B in Organic Chemistry than for that A in Advanced Anthropological Debates. Do not try to pad your GPA by taking less challenging courses or by taking only a few demanding courses at a time. Admissions committees have been doing this for a while, and are wise to such tactics. Because the PharmD curriculum is rigorous and demanding, many schools of pharmacy will evaluate your undergraduate course load closely, paying attention to the difficulty of the courses taken each term and the total credit load per term. They want applicants who have consistently carried a minimum of 14–16 credits/units per term and have performed well. (Exception: A course load of 12–14 credits is recommended for the first semester of collegiate study because this is considered the semester you transition from high school to college.) This demonstrates that you have the stamina to keep up with the full-time pharmacy course demands. Remember, good scholarship is very important and is considered a predictor for success in the pharmacy curriculum. Thus, specific evaluation of all classes will be taken into consideration along with your science GPA and overall cumulative GPA.

The admissions committee also considers grade inflation, which is prevalent at many schools. Committee members usually know which institutions tend to inflate and which don't, and they take that into account when evaluating your GPA. If your undergraduate school uses narrative course evaluations or a pass/fail system rather than letter grades, contact the admissions office of the school to which you're applying to determine if this is acceptable. Because this type of evaluation is not always a straightforward process, consider requesting a letter grade instead of just an evaluation. This is especially important for prerequisite courses in math and the sciences where a letter grade is almost always expected. Remember, if you have any personal extenuating or unique circumstances that may have influenced your academic performance, be sure to address them in your application.

As we previously noted, some pharmacy schools consider a positive trend in your GPA over time. If you got off to a slow start but have improved significantly in later semesters, you are in a favorable situation. However, if your grades have been dropping, this may be a problem and may reflect your inability to handle a demanding curriculum over time. Bottom line: The admissions committee is looking for sustained improvement over time (or, ideally, stellar marks right from the beginning!). Finally, the admissions committee will evaluate each applicant's credentials not only individually, but also in comparison with the credentials of all other applicants.

Pharmacy College Admission Test Scores

Schools recognize that the PCAT is a standardized exam that can be used as an objective, qualitative tool to help them evaluate applicants as fairly as possible. While different colleges have classes and requirements of varying difficulty, every student takes the same exact PCAT. With this test, students start on a level playing field. Keep in mind, however, that the scores are viewed only as an indicator of content retention and are not used solely as a final parameter for acceptance or nonacceptance. Remember also that some schools do not require you to take the PCAT.

With that said, while some schools set the minimum required PCAT score for admission at the 50th percentile, that score is not competitive based on recent applicant pools. Most pharmacy schools recommend that competitive applicants have PCAT scores greater than the 70th percentile composite score. Each of the five components of the PCAT is also reviewed, and average scores in each area should be 70 percent or greater. Be advised that the average PCAT score for some institutions is actually higher than 70 percent. For example, one institution reported that the admitted Fall 2006 class had PCAT scores at the 85th percentile.

Applicants must submit one set of PCAT scores. However, if you submit two or more sets of PCAT scores, the committee will view all sets but will use the highest set when considering your application for admission. If your PCAT scores are not stunning after your first test results, you may take the test again, but make sure you prepare well before you take the test a second time, especially if your test results indicate a weak area. Taking the test more than once can work in your favor if you improve the second time around.

Importance of the Interview

After a preliminary assessment of the applicant pool and review of the applicants' GPAs, PCAT scores, and personal statements (and the supplemental applications), the most qualified applicants are then invited for an on-site interview. Offers of interview are dependent upon the size and competitiveness of the applicant pool. An invitation to interview at any pharmacy school means that you're acceptable on paper and that the school would now like to get to know you in person and see if you are the stellar candidate you presented on paper. Sometimes, an applicant may appear stunning on paper (great academics and PCAT score, and motivated in his or her personal statement); however, this motivation is lacking or not conveyed at all during the interview process. Sometimes, there is a disconnect between the applicant on paper and the applicant in person. Schools are worrisome of admitting such students. Because of this, we strongly emphasize that you prepare well for your interview. Essentially, the interview is an indication of how important admissions committees believe personal characteristics are in the making of a great pharmacist.

After your interview, your interviewers will make their recommendation to the admissions committee by submitting a written statement concerning their assessment of your candidacy for pharmacy school in general and for their pharmacy program in particular. At some institutions, the interview has the potential to become the deciding factor in your admission to the school. At other schools, it is only one of the several components that factor into the overall process. This is usually the case for schools that conduct blind (or closed-file) interviews. This means that the person or team who interviews you has not reviewed your application and therefore does not know anything about you. Most pharmacy schools would agree that a particularly strong interview may ensure your acceptance.

With that said, if you had a poor interview, does that mean you will almost certainly be rejected? It depends. Remember that your interview may consist of two parts: an oral interview and a written portion. Schools that use a rule-based system (in which each portion of the application is scored separately) will factor your interview score (both oral and written) into your overall score, which means that you may still have a chance to be admitted if your overall score is high enough. On the other hand, if you really performed horribly on your interview, the admissions committee will most certainly scrutinize what happened and weigh in on the comments provided by the interviewers. Therefore, do not take the interview segment lightly. Again, we cannot overemphasize enough how important it is for you to come to your interview well prepared and focused on the ultimate goal of showing the interviewers just how much you want to attend their pharmacy school.

THE ADMISSIONS COMMITTEE: UNDERSTANDING THE PROCESS

The admissions process and the composition of the committee members vary from institution to institution. At most pharmacy schools, the majority of the admissions committee members are members of the faculty from either the clinical or basic science department and may include associate dean representatives from the Office of the Dean. Some schools also have one or more pharmacy student members representing each level of the professional classes. The primary function of the admissions committee is to review all applications for admission to the professional program and to recommend the admission of qualified applicants. All admissions committee members share in the responsibility of selecting the applicants for admission.

Upon completion of the interviews, each candidate's entire application undergoes review. While there are many different ways in which admissions committees arrive at their final decisions, there are some relatively common approaches. One approach involves the open discussion of applications during a meeting of the committee. Following the discussion of the application, the committee members may vote or assign a score to the applicant, with the applicants receiving the highest scores being admitted. Advocates of this method believe that the open discussion of applications is essential to arriving at the best decisions. Opponents argue that a particularly vocal committee member can skew the votes of the others and have an undue influence on the decision process.

> **Stand Out in the Crowd**
>
> "After chairing an admissions committee for several years, the first thing we are looking for is diversity. Not simply gender and ethnic diversity, but more importantly, a mix of backgrounds and prior experiences."
>
> —Gary, pharmacy school admissions committee member

Some admissions committees use a predetermined point system to score each component of the application where points are awarded for each part of the application (GPA, PCAT scores, interview, personal statement, letters of recommendation, experience, etc.). Candidates are then ranked on a tiered system, and those applicants with the highest scores are admitted. Advocates of this system point to the inherent fairness of treating each part of the application in the same way for all applicants. Opponents say that it minimizes the judgment each committee member can bring to the process and eliminates valuable discussion between committee members.

Schools using a holistic approach have several members of the committee read and score the application as a whole. Each reader brings his own knowledge, experience, and judgment to the process. Schools using this method believe that because the reader has access to the entire application and the freedom to score the application as a whole, he can judge the file as a whole. Each application is usually reviewed by several committee members. The use of multiple readers adds collective judgment to the evaluation of applications. Supporters of this approach value the collective judgment aspect, the opportunity for committee members to weigh the parts of applications differently depending on circumstances and to thoroughly review all application parts. Opponents point out the danger of inconsistently weighing criteria and the absence of discussion as weaknesses of this method.

Some schools may use a combination of the above approaches, such as scoring each section of the application first, followed by a committee meeting to discuss the entire application, and finally an overall vote to determine whether the applicant is accepted or not.

SHARING OF ADMISSION DECISIONS

PharmCAS institutions will receive reports regarding the number of offers of admission made and number of offers of admission accepted for those applicants the college or school shares with another PharmCAS institution. Your designated PharmCAS institutions will know how many offers of admission you have received and how many offers of admission you have accepted at other PharmCAS institutions. PharmCAS institutions will not know how many applications you have submitted in total. They will also not know whether you were denied admission to another pharmacy school, nor will they be informed of any other admission actions made by other PharmCAS institutions other than offers of admission made or accepted.

ALTERNATE LISTS

The number of applicants offered admission each year depends on the admissions numbers for each institution. The admission process is highly competitive and is dependent upon the number of applications received and the qualifications of the applicant pool. Applicants who are not offered acceptance may be placed on an alternate (waiting) list.

How an individual pharmacy school uses its alternate list is largely influenced by its acceptance policies. All pharmacy schools ultimately need to accept more students than are reflected in the actual class size. This is because many successful applicants receive multiple acceptances and therefore have to turn down all but one school, leaving the rejected schools to offer new acceptances. Admissions committees have a historical perspective as to how many acceptances they must offer to fill the pharmacy school class. Depending on the school's admissions policies, there are two basic ways alternate lists may be utilized. In the first, the dean of admissions may send out enough acceptances to initially fill the class, and wait for withdrawals to occur before sending out additional acceptances. Interviewed applicants are constantly added to the list after they clear the admissions committee, while accepted applicants are skimmed off the top. Under this process, movement on the alternate list is fluid, with applicants constantly drawn from the pool to fill openings as they occur. In the second method, the dean of admissions may decide to accept most if not all of those applicants that the admissions committee finds to be immediately acceptable, even if it results in the potential overfilling of the class. This is because the school already anticipates how many will actually accept the offer. In this case, the dean waits for an opening to occur before new offers of acceptance are made to people on the alternate list. The alternate list is used as a large holding category for the applicants who are not accepted with the initial round of acceptees.

Moreover, these two basic methods are further complicated by the fact that some pharmacy schools rank applicants on the alternate list, while others do not. A ranked waiting list of students will be established and these applicants will be notified of an offer of admission as space becomes available. Spaces in the entering class become available as admitted applicants decline their offers, usually for personal reasons or the school withdraws the offer because the applicant has not fulfilled all of the requirements for admission. For schools that do not rank the alternate list, after the deadline has passed for admitted applicants to accept and secure their spot, the committee meets again to assess how many spaces are open and reviews everyone on the waitlist to determine who will fill the space.

Unfortunately, most pharmacy schools are somewhat reluctant to discuss an applicant's chances of being accepted from the waiting list. This may be because it is impossible to predict when accepted applicants will decline the offer or be canceled, or it may be due to the fact that no one really knows how many applicants will be accepted from the alternate list in any given year. The waitlist usually will remain active until the first day of classes in the fall. Applicants who were waitlisted but did not subsequently receive an offer of admission must complete the entire application process again. Due to limits on enrollment, institutions cannot admit all qualified applicants.

CHAPTER 13

Rejection and Your Alternatives

Ultimately, there will be students who are not offered acceptance into a school of pharmacy due to the highly competitive nature of the admissions process. In fact, some admissions committees admit that qualified students are denied at their particular institution because there simply aren't enough available spaces. If you only take one piece of advice from this chapter, let it be this: If you are rejected from pharmacy school the first time around, that shouldn't stop you from applying at least a second time. Many schools would agree that reapplication is strongly encouraged.

WHAT WENT WRONG?

Before investing the time, energy, and money it takes to reapply, you need to identify those areas of your application that need improving. This involves taking the following steps:

Talk to Your Prepharmacy Advisor

Your advisor is the person most likely to have a good sense of your credentials and how they compare to those of applicants from your college who have been successful in getting into pharmacy school in the past. Your advisor may also be able to suggest reapplication strategies that other students have used successfully in the past.

Check with the Pharmacy School That Rejected You

Many pharmacy schools will give you the opportunity to talk to someone from the admissions office about your application. In particular, try to contact schools that interviewed you to find out if they will discuss aspects of your application that the admissions committee found to be weak. The admissions staff should be able to discuss its school's needs for the incoming class and how your application fits into the big picture. Keep in mind that the admissions committee at each institution dictates its own admissions policies. Therefore, what one admissions committee is looking for in a potential pharmacy student can be different from what another pharmacy school is looking for. After getting feedback from the schools you've applied to, summarize their comments and figure out how you can improve your application credentials. In general, you should be looking for those aspects of your application that most pharmacy schools believed needed strengthening.

According to some pharmacy admissions committees, the following were some easily fixable reasons that contributed to students being denied admission to their programs:

- Incomplete applications
- Missed deadlines
- A failure to follow application directions
- Did not meet the minimum requirements

The points on the above list, which were reported by many pharmacy schools, are all items that can easily be avoided the second time around. The best thing you can do to remain competitive is to thoroughly research the program of the pharmacy school you are interested in applying to well in advance. Following directions regarding deadlines and procedures is key to successfully completing your application. Check that your timing of the PCAT exam corresponds with the school's deadlines. Make sure your prerequisites are complete or will be completed before the start date of classes.

A Rebuilding Year

Take advantage of the coming year to increase your chances of success in the future by making your application even more competitive. This can be done by taking extra coursework to enhance your GPA or studying for the PCAT to improve your initial test score. If you were lacking in the extracurricular activities department, it would be helpful to involve yourself in the field of pharmacy through student membership in a professional organization, holding an office of a student organization, or volunteering or working in a pharmacy. Reevaluate your personal statement and make sure that you express yourself clearly so that the admissions committee member reading your statement will get to know something about you as a person and why you want to be a pharmacist.

Your passion for pharmacy should shine through. Finally, if you were not invited for any interviews, this may be an indication that your application did not pass the initial screening round and that it is not competitive enough to warrant an interview. On the other hand, if you did interview but did not perform well, try to figure out ways to improve next time. Perhaps you need to work on being better prepared for answering the questions by doing your research about the school's program and staying abreast of current events in the field.

> **Real-World Experience**
>
> "I advise students that if they don't get in on their first application, then continue to take classes, but gain some experience in the field either working as a technician in a pharmacy or as a laboratory assistant in a research laboratory."
>
> —Howard, pharmacy school admissions counselor

Better Timing the Second Time Around

If you applied late to a pharmacy school that admits students on a rolling admissions and you interviewed in the last round, it is likely that your rejection was related to poor timing. Reapply the next chance you get, making sure to get your completed application out as early as possible. It is also possible that you didn't get accepted because you applied to the wrong schools. Go over your list with your advisor to be sure you are applying to those schools that will look at your application in the most positive light.

> **Improving Your Chances**
>
> To improve your chances of acceptance the second time around:
>
> - Retake courses.
> - Retake the PCAT.
> - Reconsider your timing.
> - Rethink your school selection.

POSTBACCALAUREATE PROGRAMS

Postbaccalaureate (post-bac) programs are academic programs specifically designed to help applicants improve their chances of gaining admissions to health profession schools. Specifically, some universities offer the Post-Bac Pre-Health Professions Program to students who already have a BS or BA degree in any subject but who need additional science courses to meet admission requirements for health profession schools, such as pharmacy school. Students who want to increase their chance of admission to the school of their choice by improving their academic credentials (because they have earned marginal grades in the sciences and need to strengthen their academic record) will also benefit from the program.

Pharmacy-Specific Post-Bac Programs

Post-bac programs are usually designed to prepare students to apply to any health profession. However, there are some programs that are specific to prepare students for certain schools, such as medical school or pharmacy school. The **LECOM School of Pharmacy Post Baccalaureate Program** is one program that is specifically tailored to prepare students for continuing studies toward a PharmD degree at any accredited pharmacy school. This program will introduce pharmaceutical sciences to students to prepare and enhance their knowledge of the discipline. While this program does provide an opportunity for the student to demonstrate academic capability, its successful completion does not guarantee admission to the LECOM School of Pharmacy or any other Doctor of Pharmacy program. For more information on this program, visit its website at www.lecom.edu/pharm/application/pharm-post-bac.asp. Most pharmacy schools that offer post-bac studies are only for those individuals who already have a BS Pharm and are now returning for a PharmD.

CONSIDER THE ALTERNATIVES

As you already know, getting into pharmacy school is not a simple task. It involves careful planning, time, and energy to repeat the application cycle. If pharmacy is your passion, by all means reapply to give yourself another shot at your dreams of becoming a pharmacist. Remember, however, to only tackle the reapplication process with a marked improvement in your credentials.

If you're having doubts, be sure to reevaluate your initial decision of wanting to go into the field. Begin by assessing your reasons for pursuing a career in pharmacy. What drew you to the idea of becoming a pharmacist? Was it a desire to help people? A love of science and problem solving? The intellectual challenge? Or something else? Knowing the answers to these questions can help you to start investigating other professions that may provide you with the same rewards and challenges. Do you want a career in the health professions or will another area, such as research or teaching, meet your needs? If you are really more interested in research, find out what area of study fascinates you most. If you enjoy pharmaceutical research, then perhaps pursuing a graduate career in this area would be more relevant and bring you one step closer to your goal of being a researcher. Taking the time to figure out your true passion and to redefine your career path now will benefit you in the long run because you will then be doing what you love and enjoy in life.

PART FOUR

Preparing for Your Career in Pharmacy

CHAPTER 14

What to Expect and Do in Pharmacy School

You'll learn the nuts and bolts of what you need to know to be a pharmacist in pharmacy school, but some of the most important aspects of your learning can take place outside of the classroom. While in pharmacy school, you should take the opportunity to be involved in school and community activities. We encourage you to be an active student pharmacist by taking part in student organizations and fraternities, and by participating in local community events such as health fairs.

ORGANIZATIONS WITHIN PHARMACY SCHOOLS

There are numerous organizations for students in pharmacy school. Some are social. Three pharmaceutical fraternities—Kappa Epsilon, Kappa Psi, and Phi Delta Chi—and one national pharmacy leadership society—Phi Lambda Sigma—are linked with most schools of pharmacy. Others are professional, nationally recognized organizations— American Pharmacists Association (APhA), American College of Clinical Pharmacy, International Society of Pharmaceutical Engineering, American Association of Pharmaceutical Science, National Community Pharmacists Association, and the American Society of Hospital Systems (ASHP)—that have student chapters or membership. There is also the Academy of Students of Pharmacy. In addition, the APhA and ASHP usually have state chapters. The International Pharmaceutical Students Federation (IPSF) is a worldwide federation of student pharmacist organizations whose goal is to encourage cooperation to improve the profession of pharmacy.

It is in your best interest to be active in some of these groups because membership in these student organizations entitles you to a variety of programs, services, and resources. You may attend professional educational programs on disease state management (DSM) or health issue updates and pharmacy conferences (usually at a reduced program registration fee), and you can usually become politically involved with the profession's policies at all levels of government. You will also be able to network with peers and mentors as well as obtain leadership experience. Some organizations offer complimentary subscriptions to their respective official journals or publications and special discounts on many required pharmacy textbooks and references. More importantly, a few organizations offer guidance on professional, leadership, and career development. No matter which organization you decide to join, we believe that membership in one will no doubt enhance your education, help you explore careers in pharmacy through their career network, and keep you connected with others in the profession.

In addition to these professional organizations, there is one academic honor society in pharmacy, the Rho Chi Society, which lets you graduate with honors distinction. Admission to this organization is based on the grade point average (GPA) within your professional program recognizing students for their outstanding scholastic achievement.

WORKING WHILE IN SCHOOL

Clearly academics are your first priority in school—you want to maintain a solid GPA and comprehend as much in class as possible. However, part-time work during pharmacy school is possible. In fact, some believe those individuals who work in the pharmacy during their professional education do better in school and comprehend more because those students are comfortable with the drug names, the issues surrounding retail or hospital pharmacy work, and the mathematical calculations that are often associated with the pharmacy profession.

As a pharmacy student, you will be able to apply for a pharmacy intern license, which allows you to engage in the practice of pharmacy under the supervision of a pharmacist. The board of pharmacy for each state has specific guidelines on issuing the intern license to students actively working toward the requirements for licensure as a pharmacist (i.e., you must be enrolled in a pharmacy program). With this intern license, you may work as an intern while gaining exposure to different types of pharmacy practices, giving you the opportunity to explore the different career pathways available to you after graduation.

INTERNSHIPS

During summer breaks, we encourage you to take advantage of the internships that are made available through various government agencies, pharmaceutical companies, community chain drug stores, and professional organizations. Taking part in these internships will help you have a better perspective of the different career paths that a PharmD degree can offer. This will also give you an opportunity to explore whether you are interested in these various positions.

Most of the internships are paid and may provide some sort of housing assistance. These are usually short-term internships (about 12 weeks long) beginning mid-May and ending mid-August. They are intensively structured and are designed to provide students the chance to gain invaluable experience within a specific practice area. Because these internships are highly sought after and depend on the number of available openings each year, the selection process may be competitive. Final decisions are usually based on GPA, communication skills, and leadership abilities.

Use internships to help build your career while you're still in school. For example, if you have an interest in the pharmaceutical industry, you may want to consider participating in an internship program that offers industry experience to gain knowledge and insight into one of the following departments: regulatory affairs, research and development, sales and marketing, or medical/clinical affairs. Throughout an internship, students work on specific projects, gain a perspective of opportunities for pharmacists in the industry setting, and even learn what it is really like to be an employee of a major pharmaceutical company. Internship programs like these introduce participants to company principles, challenge them to think creatively, and provide hands-on experience that will help prepare them for a career in healthcare.

Some retail pharmacy chains (e.g., Walgreens, Rite-Aid) offer either summer pharmacy internships in their stores or corporate internships at their corporate headquarters to allow students to learn more about the corporate operations of a retail chain. The Academy of Managed Care Pharmacy *(www.amcp.org)* provides a listing of internships available to pharmacy students in areas such as managed care, hospital pharmacy, and association management. If you would like more information on the vast opportunities that exist in professional organizations and learn about their policies and management, you can inquire about the internship programs that are available from national pharmacy associations such as the National Community Pharmacists Association (NCPA), APhA, or ASHP.

Keep in mind that you will also have the opportunity to explore these various career options in pharmacy during the experiential component of your pharmacy curriculum. These clinical/pharmacy practice rotations are usually six to eight weeks long (again depending on the institution) and constitute a mandatory requirement to your PharmD degree. Consult with your school on specific requirements for this experiential training period.

PREPARING FOR THE LICENSE EXAM (NAPLEX)

Upon graduation, you will need to acquire a license to practice pharmacy, which is required in all states, the District of Columbia, and all U.S. territories. To obtain a license, you need to serve an internship under a licensed pharmacist, graduate from an accredited college of pharmacy, and pass an examination. After earning a pharmacy degree, successful graduates go on to take the NAPLEX, or North American Pharmacist Licensure Examination, which is the national board examination that tests the pharmacy skills and knowledge required to become a registered pharmacist. All states require the NAPLEX and 45 states and the District of Columbia also require the Multistate Pharmacy Jurisprudence Exam (MPJE), which tests pharmacy law (more on the MPJE in the next section). Pharmacists in the states that do not require the MJPE must past a state-specific exam that is similar to the MJPE. In addition to the NAPLEX and MPJE, some states require additional tests unique to their state and some have a separate pharmacy exam altogether. Pharmacists can apply for certification in multiple states and often do not need to retest in order to use their license elsewhere if they want to move. You will need to contact the board of pharmacy in the state you are seeking licensure for more information on examination requirements and license transfer procedures.

During your fourth year of pharmacy school, you will start studying for your license exam. The best way to approach your preparation is to get your hands on as many sample tests and questions as you can. Working through sample questions or practice exam questions will help you gain confidence with the test format as your time for testing approaches.

About the NAPLEX

The NAPLEX is developed by the National Association of Boards of Pharmacy (NABP) and is utilized by the state boards of pharmacy as part of their assessment of competence to practice pharmacy. The test is designed to assess your knowledge and ability in pharmacy. By using the NAPLEX, the state boards provide a valid and objective examination that tests competence in important aspects of the practice of pharmacy. The NAPLEX also assists the state boards of pharmacy in fulfilling one aspect of their responsibility to safeguard public health and welfare. To register for the NAPLEX, contact the board of pharmacy in the state from which you are seeking licensure for a registration form. If you are currently enrolled in a pharmacy program, your school should provide you with the necessary information during the fourth year of your attendance on the application procedure. You may also register online at *www.nabp.net*.

What's on the NAPLEX Exam?

The NAPLEX is a computer-adaptive examination that consists of 185 multiple-choice test questions. Of these, 150 questions will be used to calculate your test score and the remaining 35 items will serve as pretest questions, which are dispersed throughout the examination and (try as you might) cannot be identified by the test taker. The pretest questions will not affect your NAPLEX score but are used to evaluate the item's difficulty level for possible inclusion as a scored question in future examinations.

A majority of the questions on the NAPLEX are asked in a scenario-based format (i.e., patient profiles with accompanying test questions). To properly analyze and answer the questions presented, you must refer to the information provided in the patient profile. Other questions are answered solely from the information provided in the question.

What Is the Pre-NAPLEX?

The Pre-NAPLEX is a practice examination to help familiarize you with the NAPLEX testing experience. It is the only NAPLEX practice examination written and developed by the NABP and is not intended for use as a study guide. Rather, it is designed as a practice test to get you comfortable with the actual exam. The Pre-NAPLEX will benefit those who are preparing for the NAPLEX by exhibiting the same look and feel as the actual licensure examination as well as providing a score estimate. Taking the Pre-NAPLEX will give you the chance to "preview" the NAPLEX experience before exam day. For detailed information on the Pre-NAPLEX, visit the NABP website.

MULTISTATE PHARMACY JURISPRUDENCE EXAM (MPJE)

Most states require a pharmacy drug law examination as a condition of licensure. The Multistate Pharmacy Jurisprudence Examination (MPJE) is currently administered in 45 U.S. jurisdictions. An applicant may register to take the NAPLEX and MPJE at the same time upon meeting all eligibility requirements. The MPJE is a two-hour, computer-adaptive test that combines federal- and state-specific law questions to serve as the state law examination in participating jurisdictions. Questions on the MPJE are tailored to the specific laws in each state and candidates must take a separate exam for each state or jurisdiction in which they are seeking licensure. The MPJE consists of 90 multiple-choice test questions: 60 questions will be used to calculate the test score, and the remaining 30 items serve as pretest questions which do affect the MPJE score. Like in the NAPLEX, the pretest questions are dispersed throughout the examination and cannot be identified by the candidate.

CHAPTER 15

Postprofessional (Post-PharmD)– Residencies, Fellowships, and Board Certifications

After you receive your PharmD, your career path can head in several different directions. Upon graduating from pharmacy school, some students may choose to complete a residency and/or fellowship to enhance their pharmacy training, while others may choose to pursue further graduate study.

RESIDENCIES

A pharmacy residency is a directed, postgraduate training in a defined area of pharmacy practice. It provides the knowledge and experience that pharmacy practitioners need to face today's complex healthcare environment, while also providing essential skills to meet the practice demands of the constantly evolving profession. In recent years, there has been an increasing number of students seeking residency training in pharmacy practice. With more than 800 pharmacy residency programs available in hospitals, community pharmacies and some specialized facilities, the options are endless. These residency programs are offered in general pharmacy practice, clinical pharmacy practice, community pharmacies, ambulatory care settings, and other specialty areas to match your personal interests and specific career requirements. In some cases, completion of a pharmacy residency is sometimes a requirement for employment in a hospital clinical pharmacy practice setting or in clinical faculty positions at pharmacy schools.

Why a Residency?

The purpose of a pharmacy residency is to prepare pharmacists for practice. Residencies are also the best way for pharmacists to learn more about a specialized area of interest. They primarily train pharmacists in professional practice and management activities and provide experience in integrating pharmacy services with the comprehensive needs of individual practice settings. The in-depth experiences you receive results in the attainment of advanced practice skills and knowledge.

Residency training offers many benefits, including a competitive advantage in the job market, networking opportunities, and career planning. Many employers recognize the value of residency training because the intense one-year residency experience is often considered equivalent to two to three years of work experience. Thus, those who have completed a residency have an advantage over those who have not in terms of the years of pharmacy practice experience. Opportunities are there for residents to expand their network of professional contacts and to explore different practice settings. Many programs can arrange for residents to visit other residency programs or to complete a portion of their residency at another practice site. During the course of training, residents will be able to better determine their interest in a particular area of pharmacy practice. While residents earn a modest salary (as compared to the typical pharmacist's salary), the experience they gain during their training is invaluable to their professional development.

Types of Residencies

There are two types of residencies. PGY1 (Post-Graduate Year 1) residencies provide training for general pharmacy practice in health systems, managed care, or community settings. PGY2 (Post-Graduate Year 2) residencies provide advanced training in a specialized area of patient care (discussed below). Pharmacies within hospitals differ considerably from community pharmacies and thus require a different set of practice skills. Some pharmacists in hospital pharmacies may have more complex clinical medication management issues whereas pharmacists in community pharmacies often have more complex business and customer-relations issues. Because of the complexity of medications including specific indications, effectiveness of treatment regimens, safety of medications (i.e., drug interactions), and patient compliance issues (in the hospital and at home), many pharmacists practicing in hospitals gain more education and training after pharmacy school through a pharmacy practice residency, which is sometimes followed by another specialized residency in a specific area. Those pharmacists are referred to as clinical pharmacists and often times become specialized in various disciplines of pharmacy. For example, these subspecialties include hematology/oncology, HIV/AIDS, infectious disease, critical care, emergency medicine, toxicology, nuclear pharmacy, pain management, psychiatry, anticoagulation clinics, pediatrics/neonatal pharmacy, and more. After completing a PGY1 residency in general practice, some pharmacists continue to the second-year and more specialized PGY2 residency or enter into a fellowship.

Researching Residencies

You can find out information on residencies by going to the American Society of Health-System Pharmacists (ASHP) Residency Directory site at www.ashp.org for ASHP-accredited residency programs. The ASHP accreditation standard provides criteria that every residency program must meet in order to receive and maintain accreditation. As part of the accreditation standards, each resident is required to complete a residency project and present the findings at a regional residency conference, known as the Western States Resident's Conference, held yearly in Monterey, California. The ASHP directory lists all accredited hospital and institutional residencies. You can search by institution name, state, pharmacy practice residencies, or specialized residency program to get a list of pharmacy residencies programs. The Residency Program Showcase at the ASHP Midyear Clinical Meeting is an event that gives students and pharmacists a chance to talk with representatives from a wide range of residencies. The ASHP Resident Matching Program is a service that matches applicants with residencies according to the preferences of each. To plan your residency experience, visit the *CareerPharm* website at *www.careerpharm.com*, maintained by the ASHP, which provides useful resources and information on how to select the right residency program for you. ASHP also publishes the document, "Why Should I do a Residency?" which provides insights about pharmacy residency training and suggests a timeline for applying during the last year of school (this is also available on the ASHP website).

The American College of Clinical Pharmacy (ACCP) Directory of Residencies and Fellowships *(www.accp.com)* describes more than 200 residencies and fellowships being offered that can be referenced by state and by practice/research specialty. The Academy of Managed Care Pharmacy *(www.amcp.org)* provides a listing of the available managed care residencies nationwide while the American Pharmacists Association *(www.aphanet.org)* provides a listing for community pharmacy residency programs.

FELLOWSHIPS

A pharmacy fellowship is a directed, highly individualized, postgraduate training program designed to prepare the participant to become an independent researcher. In contrast to a residency, which places emphasis on the development of practice skills, a fellowship is focused on the development of research skills. Fellowships are designed to primarily develop competency in the scientific research process, including conceptualizing, planning, conducting, and reporting research. The goal is to prepare highly motivated participants to become independent researchers. There are opportunities to take graduate coursework and to participate in clinical and laboratory investigations with experienced clinical and basic science faculty. Fellows participate in ongoing, funded research as well as in the design and conduct of original research under the guidance of a preceptor. Completion of this program prepares the trainee for tenure-track academic and research scientist positions. A listing of available fellowships can be found on the ACCP website.

TRAINING AND CAREER DEVELOPMENT FOR PHARMD RESEARCHERS

The National Institutes of Health (NIH) recognizes that PharmD's contribute to the health of society through education, patient care, and research, and that their knowledge of drug therapies is important for virtually all human diseases.

As such, the NIH has created a website (*www.nigms.nih.gov/Training/PharmD*) to provide information about NIH funding opportunities for PharmD students, post-doctoral researchers, and faculty interested in biomedical and behavioral research. Resources available through this gateway include information about grant-writing tips and research training opportunities, as well as career development awards and resources.

GRADUATE STUDY

You also have the opportunity to complete advanced study (such as graduate work for a master of science [MS] or doctor of philosophy [PhD] degree) at many colleges of pharmacy. Graduate study can be pursued in any of the specialized areas of pharmacy such as pharmacology, toxicology, pharmaceutics, pharmacoeconomics, or regulatory science. PharmD graduates who pursue this route often times decide that they would like to pursue an academic career as a professor, focusing their research on any one of the above subspecialties. Other pharmacists interested in public policy usually pursue a master's or PhD degree in Public Health or Health Policy. Still others may pursue an MBA for a career in pharmacy operations, in healthcare management, or for entrepreneurial purposes.

BOARD CERTIFICATIONS

Pharmacists may choose to specialize in one of six areas and receive board certification in any of them. The value of board certification demonstrates to society (and the patient) that an individual pharmacy specialist possesses a high level of expertise in a particular area of pharmacy specialty. While board certification may provide a competitive edge in obtaining jobs and in job retention with an increase in pay, it definitely makes the job even more challenging to any pharmacist who wants to specialize in a particular area. To recognize specialty areas of pharmacy practice, the American Pharmacists Association (APhA) created the Board of Pharmacy Specialties (BPS) in 1976. The goal of this board is to protect public health by verifying the level of training, knowledge, and skills of pharmacists in recognized areas of specialty practice. BPS offers certification in the following specialties: Nuclear Pharmacy, Nutrition Support Pharmacy, Oncology Pharmacy, Pharmacotherapy, Psychiatric Pharmacy, and Ambulatory Care Pharmacy.

> **Get on Board**
>
> "Board certification is a seal of accomplishments. I took the BCPS boards several years ago and found them fair, but challenging. As a manager hiring pharmacists at this point in my career, simply having a license is a minimum, but having board credentials tells me this person is motivated."
>
> —Nilou, graduate of University of Southern California

Pharmacists must meet a set of requirements, which include specific educational and experience-based criteria as well as passing an exam, to be certified in one of these specialties. For more information on board certification, interested individuals may contact the BPS website at www.bps.org. These BPS certification programs are accredited by the National Commission for Certifying Agencies (NCCA), the accrediting body of the National Organization for Competency Assurance. BPS joins an elite group of organizations with programs that have received and maintained the prestigious NCCA accreditation. BPS is the only organization that certifies pharmacists to achieve this distinction.

Nuclear Pharmacy

This discipline seeks to improve and promote health through the safe and effective use of radioactive drugs for diagnosis and therapy. Nuclear pharmacy (sometimes referred to as radiopharmacy) involves the compounding and dispensing of radioactive materials for use in nuclear imaging and nuclear medical procedures. Nuclear imaging offers a safe and reliable alternative to invasive diagnostic procedures and surgery, and is used to assess the structure and function of organs such as the kidneys, liver, lungs, brain, or heart. Nuclear pharmacists compound radioactive pharmaceuticals for diagnostic purposes—for example, compounding radioactive products for diagnosing heart function. The nuclear pharmacist will dispense the prepared product to the nuclear medicine department of a clinic or hospital where the dose will be administered to the patient.

> ### Above and Beyond
>
> "I expect the pharmacists working for me to stay abreast of current trends in healthcare. Sure they all get 15 hours of continuing education, but I want them to be at the cutting edge of pharmacotherapy through other avenues (attending meetings, taking BCPS review courses, etc.)."
>
> —Nancy, graduate of University of Michigan

Nutrition Support Pharmacy

This discipline addresses the care of patients with potential or existing nutritional problems caused by illness, surgery, or other conditions. The nutrition support pharmacist is responsible for performing nutritional assessments and developing patient-specific nutritional regimens for patients who have special digestion concerns and critical dosing requirements. These specialists will monitor patients who are receiving nutrition support therapy (such as parenteral and enteral nutrition) to ensure that optimal nutritional support is maintained and evaluate the effect of the patient's nutrition status on drug therapy.

Oncology Pharmacy

The oncology pharmacist is a specialist on the treatment team for patients with cancer and plays an important role in managing and preventing cancer- and treatment-related complications. Because chemotherapy and related cancer treatments are extremely complex and vital, working with cancer patients and their doctors can be a challenging yet rewarding career path for these pharmacy specialists. They are considered the experts in the pharmacology and optimal use of cancer chemotherapy, and practice in a variety of acute and outpatient treatment centers that involve the care of cancer patients, including those undergoing bone marrow transplantations. The oncology pharmacist provides information about chemotherapy medications, determines optimal drug dosing of these agents, and helps develop treatment guidelines to ensure the optimal use of chemotherapy drugs and supportive therapies.

Pharmacotherapy

This discipline involves ensuring the safe, appropriate, and economical use of drugs in patient care. A pharmacotherapy specialist can be considered a generalist pharmacy practitioner (or pharmacy's equivalent to internal medicine) who has demonstrated a mastery of knowledge and skills in a broad range of pharmacotherapy topics. The pharmacotherapy specialist is responsible for direct patient care, functions as an integral member of a multidisciplinary healthcare team, and is recognized as an expert in the area of applied pharmacotherapeutics. The specialist possesses advanced-level experience, training, and skills in the area of biomedical, pharmaceutical, and clinical sciences, and practices in a variety of settings including health systems, academia, and the pharmaceutical industry.

Psychiatric Pharmacy

This discipline involves the pharmaceutical care of patients with psychiatric-related illnesses. Complex mental conditions require the use of psychotropics, or psychiatric medicines, which are commonly prescribed in most healthcare settings. The psychiatric pharmacy specialist is responsible for optimizing drug therapy for psychotropic medications, monitors patient response, assesses for drug-induced problems, and recommends appropriate treatment plans.

Ambulatory Care Pharmacy

The new specialty in ambulatory care pharmacy was approved in June 2009 and is scheduled for its first examination in 2011. This discipline involves the provision of integrated, accessible healthcare services by pharmacists through direct patient care and medication management for ambulatory patients, long-term relationships, coordination of care, and developing sustained partnerships with patients and practicing in the context of family and community. The ambulatory care pharmacists manage complex medication regimens in ambulatory patients, integrate care of acute illnesses and exacerbations in the context of chronic conditions, and coordinate care among members of the healthcare team. The specialists advocate for patient education and engage in health promotion, wellness, and self-management.

CHAPTER 16

Career Options

Diversity is key in the pharmacy profession. In this chapter, we will highlight the diverse opportunities that exist in the field. Given the numerous options available, it will be difficult for most pharmacy school graduates to decide what the most suitable position is for them. To consider a potential career path, the most important question to ask yourself is whether you will be happy doing what you will be hired to do. You will need to determine if you have amassed the required skills throughout your work and education, and whether you will be using the skills you enjoy most. As you go through the job search process, keep in mind that there is no better satisfaction than enjoying what you are paid to do, even if it means you may be making a little less than your colleagues working in positions you decided were not the best fit for you.

At the beginning of this book, we asked you to get to know pharmacy and find out what the profession has to offer. After you have taken undergraduate and prepharm courses, taken your PCATs, applied to and attended pharmacy school, and perhaps completed a fellowship or residency, it's time to once again get to know yourself and your passions to see what you can offer to the profession for the long haul.

Pharmacy Careers is a publication published twice yearly (January and September) by ASCEND Media that provides valuable information to graduating pharmacy students on various opportunities in pharmacy. The publication is available online at www.pharmacytimes.com.

COMMUNITY PHARMACY PRACTICE

On the healthcare team, community pharmacists are the most publicly-accessible members. Nearly 6 out of every 10 pharmacists provide care to patients in a community setting. In fact, most people see their local community pharmacist and probably visit the pharmacy more often before calling upon their doctor. Community pharmacists provide counseling about preventive medicine, especially during the flu and cold season, and are a valuable resource for people seeking advice or information about medications. As part of their role in serving the community, they refer patients to other sources of help and care, such as physicians, when necessary. Because community pharmacists spend the most time educating patients and maintaining and monitoring patient records, patients have come to depend on them as a healthcare and information resource expert. It is no surprise then that pharmacists are considered one of the most trustworthy healthcare professionals.

Leadership within Community Pharmacy

If you develop a desire to combine your professional talents with the challenge of the fast-moving retail pharmacy business, then you may want to consider a management position within a chain pharmacy practice or ownership of your own pharmacy. In chain practice, career paths usually begin at the store level, with possible subsequent advancement to a position at the district, regional, or corporate level. Many chains have management development programs in marketing operations, legal affairs, third-party programs, computerization, and pharmacy affairs. Additionally, independent retail practice offers the opportunity for you to be "your own boss." Most independent pharmacists have the spirit of entrepreneurship and motivation to successfully own their own pharmacy or, through establishing consultation services, own their own pharmacy practice. For this reason, some may pursue a management degree to develop a business sense in becoming a pharmacy owner. Interested individuals should contact the National Community Pharmacists Association at *www.ncpanet.org* for available resources on independent community pharmacy.

CONSULTANT PHARMACY AND SENIOR CARE PHARMACY

Consultant pharmacists manage and review medication regimens and supply pharmacy products and services to patients being cared for at home or in long-term care facilities (such as nursing homes, subacute care, assisted living facilities, mental health rehabilitation centers, and correctional institutions). They evaluate drug therapies and patient profiles, inform the institution's staff of new medications, and oversee the medication distribution process. In doing so, they manage and improve drug therapy and the quality of life of the senior population residing in these living environments. "Senior care pharmacy" refers to the practice of consultant pharmacy for seniors in noninstitutional settings. Thus, senior care pharmacists in general address the healthcare needs of the senior population wherever they reside.

The focus of a consultant and senior care pharmacy practice is elderly patients because they are more likely to suffer from medication-related problems such as adverse drug events, drug interactions, excessive use of medications, and inappropriate and duplicative drug therapy. They also often face complications due to their complex medication regimens. Because of this and due to the rapid growth of the aging population, the practice of consultant and senior care pharmacy has extended beyond the elderly living in institutional settings (i.e., nursing facilities or assisted living facilities) to include seniors wherever they reside, especially those living in the community.

As such, knowledge of geriatric pharmacotherapy is a basic prerequisite to working as a consultant and senior care pharmacist. The American Society of Consultant Pharmacists (ASCP) is the international professional association that provides leadership, education, advocacy, and resources to advance the practice of consultant and senior care pharmacy. The Commission for Certification in Geriatric Pharmacy (CCGP) has a website with information about becoming a Certified Geriatric Pharmacist (CGP), offering an examination in geriatric pharmacotherapy. Over 1,300 pharmacists have successfully completed the examination and become CGPs. By becoming a CGP, along with receiving extensive geriatric training, you will obtain the necessary skills to further develop and expand the practice of pharmacy for the benefit of America's aging population. To learn more about the basics of geriatric pharmacotherapy or prepare for the CCGP examination, you can visit the most comprehensive learning site for pharmacists, *www.GeriatricPharmacyReview.com*, which was developed by the ASCP. Many pharmacists practice consultant pharmacy as a component of another practice, such as a community or hospital practice. According to the ASCP, there are approximately 10,000 pharmacists who work in this type of pharmacy setting.

HOSPITAL PHARMACY PRACTICE

Pharmacy practice in the hospital setting involves pharmacists as members of a healthcare team composed of physicians, nurses, dieticians, and other hospital professionals. This setting provides hospital pharmacists a unique opportunity for direct involvement with patient care. As a hospital pharmacist, you will utilize your knowledge and clinical skills and be relied upon as an authoritative source of drug information for physicians, nurses, and patients. In addition to direct patient care involvement, pharmacists in hospitals are responsible for drug distribution, ensuring that each patient receives the appropriate drug therapy, in the correct form and dosage, and at the correct time. Hospital pharmacists maintain records on all patients, monitor them for complex medication dosing regimens, and screen for drug allergies and adverse drug effects.

Contemporary hospital pharmacy practice is composed of a number of highly specialized areas (as we have mentioned previously) that may require advance education and training in the form of residencies or board certification. For example, hospitals provide specialized services in adult medicine, pediatrics, oncology, psychiatry, nuclear pharmacy, drug and poison information, or intravenous therapy. The nature and size of the hospital helps to determine the extent to which these specialized pharmacy services are needed and utilized.

Diverse opportunities also exist in pharmacy operations and management expertise, including finance and budgeting, personnel administration, systems development, and planning. Recently, the field of information technology (IT) has exploded, creating a high demand for such specialists in the pharmacy department to be well versed in computer-based systems—such as the computerized physician order entry (CPOE) application, which is a system that allows physicians to directly enter medication orders in the hospital computer. The CPOE system has the benefit of reducing errors by minimizing the ambiguity of hand-written orders, thereby increasing patient safety.

The American Society of Health-System Pharmacists (ASHP) is the national professional association that represents pharmacists who practice in hospitals, health maintenance organizations (HMOs), long-term care facilities, home care, and other components of the healthcare system. Approximately 38,000 registered pharmacists work on a full- or part-time basis in hospitals or nursing homes. The demand for practitioners in this area of pharmacy continues to grow as hospital pharmacists continue to become more involved in providing patient-oriented services. In fact, residencies in general pharmacy practice have increased in recent years in order to train more clinical pharmacists for hospital practice. Likewise, a basic requirement to practice as a clinical pharmacist nowadays includes completion of an ASHP-accredited residency.

MANAGED CARE PHARMACY

As society's healthcare needs evolve, there has been an increased emphasis on the provision of that care through organized managed healthcare settings. This has resulted in a dramatic growth in pharmacy services in HMOs and related organizations that offer coordinated ambulatory care services staffed by a multidisciplinary team of health professionals including pharmacists, nurse practitioners, and physician assistants. In this setting, pharmacists are heavily relied on to provide primary leadership in the development of both clinical and administrative systems to manage and improve the use of medications.

Managed care organizations (MCOs) are designed to optimize patient care and outcomes and to foster quality through greater coordination of medical services. MCOs incorporate pharmaceutical care to improve access to primary and preventive care and to ensure the most appropriate and effective use of medical services in the most cost-effective manner. Opportunities for pharmacists practicing in these types of settings are numerous, given the significant growth of the managed care system in today's society.

Managed care pharmacists can play a dynamic role within MCOs. They are often involved in practice guideline and protocol development, working directly with physicians and other caregivers to determine which medical treatments and/or drug therapies are most effective in enhancing patient outcomes and improving quality of life. This includes regularly reviewing medical literature to determine which medications are the safest and most effective for treating certain diseases, and collecting data from the plan's patient population to perform analyses based on that research. As a managed care pharmacist, you will likely be involved in drug utilization review or drug use evaluation, which involves determining which patients and prescribers are using particular medications. In essence, you are trying to figure out the physician-prescribing pattern to determine whether some patients and/or prescribers may be inappropriately prescribing or using prescription drugs.

You may also be involved with care management programs, also known as disease state management (DSM) programs. These programs involve effective management and coordination of the overall care of patients who are at high risk of serious complications because of certain disease states. For example, a care management program might identify all diabetic patients within a certain plan population. As a DSM coordinator, you will make sure that those patients receive regular education and counseling about their disease, including how and when to take their medications.

Other roles that pharmacists can assume in the managed care setting include contracting with local pharmacies (to develop networks to serve plan members); contracting with pharmaceutical manufacturers (to receive rebates on prescription drug products and other value-added services); processing claims (so patient-prescriber data can be transmitted electronically to ensure accurate claims payment and provide information to assist with clinical functions such as drug utilization review); and developing and managing the plan's formulary. The Academy of Managed Care Pharmacy is the professional association of individual pharmacists who use the tools and techniques of managed care in the practice of pharmacy.

THE PHARMACEUTICAL INDUSTRY

Another area for a career in pharmacy is the pharmaceutical industry (a position within a drug company), which produces chemicals, prescription and nonprescription drugs, and other health products. Pharmacists are involved in marketing, research and product development, quality control, sales, and administration. In order to meet the technical demands and scientific duties required in pharmaceutical manufacturing, some pharmacists have gone on to obtain postgraduate degrees. Pharmacists with an interest in sales and administration can combine this with their technical background in pharmacy by serving as a medical service representative to provide expertise on the uses and merits of the products their firms produce. Experienced and successful medical service representatives with administrative abilities often rise to supervisory or executive posts in the pharmaceutical industry. Pharmacists are also employed as sales representatives, supervisors, and administrators in wholesale drug firms. If you are interested in corporate management, you can pursue a master's degree in business and administration in order to assume a leadership role on the company's management side. According to the Pharmacy Manpower Project, approximately 2 percent of all active pharmacists' time is spent in careers within the pharmaceutical industry.

ACADEMIC PHARMACY

Pharmacists practicing in an academic setting have the responsibility to train future members of the profession and conduct research to support and improve practice. If you enjoy teaching and research, then pursuing a career in academia would be the right path to take. Working in academia usually involves little contact with patients; however, this depends on your research emphasis and the position you hold. Pharmacists in academia can have jobs in a clinical or a basic science faculty. Research may include laboratory studies such as understanding the pharmacology of investigational drugs or pharmacogenomics studies or evaluation of large amounts of data in outcomes research.

Clinical pharmacy faculty have significant responsibility for patient care in addition to teaching and research. These academicians often are called educator/practitioners, serving as role models for pharmacy students and residents in many practice settings. Basic science faculties are mainly concerned with "bench" research that includes sophisticated instrumentation and techniques, analytical methods, and animal models. Pharmacy administration research often uses survey methods and statistical analyses to solve complex problems of drug utilization management, healthcare delivery, marketing, management, and other practice issues.

Pharmacists in academic positions can be employed in pharmacy schools, medical schools, or schools that train other healthcare professionals. Over 4,500 full-time faculty members work in the nation's colleges and schools of pharmacy, and are involved with teaching, research, and public service, as well as sometimes participating in patient care. Others serve as consultants for local, state, national, and international agencies' organizations. To become a faculty member at a pharmacy institution usually requires a postgraduate degree and/or advanced training (e.g., a PhD or residency or fellowship training following the professional degree program). Given the recent growth of popularity in pharmacy schools, there is currently a national shortage of faculty, creating excellent opportunities in this setting for current pharmacy students. Academia allows you the freedom to be your own boss in terms of establishing your own research and it remains extremely important in laying the groundwork for continuing advances in the field.

GOVERNMENTAL AGENCIES

Pharmacists use their basic educational backgrounds in a host of federal and state positions. At the federal level, pharmacists hold staff and supervisory posts in the U.S. Public Health Service (PHS) (more on the PHS below), the Veterans Administration, the Food and Drug Administration (FDA), the National Institutes of Health (NIH), the Centers for Disease Control and Prevention (CDC), and in all branches of the armed services. Some of these posts provide commissioned officer status, while others fall under civil service. At the state level, there are agencies charged with regulating the practice of pharmacy to preserve and protect the public health. These legal boards governing pharmacy practice usually have pharmacists employed as full-time executive officers. Also, each state pharmacy board employs pharmacists as board inspectors. As more state health agencies consolidate their purchases, a pharmacist is often engaged as a purchaser of medical and pharmaceutical supplies for the entire state.

U.S. PUBLIC HEALTH SERVICE

One of the best kept secrets for those in pharmacy is the U.S. Public Health Service led by the Surgeon General of the United States. Along with the Army, Air Force, Navy, Marines, Coast Guard, and the National Oceanographic and Atmospheric Administration, the PHS rounds out the seven uniformed services. The PHS Commissioned Corps offers a variety of employment opportunities for professionals throughout the Department of Health and Human Services (HHS) and certain non-HHS federal agencies/programs. Commissioned Corps officer status provides opportunities for mobility, flexibility, and career advancement in diverse work settings.

PHS offers two opportunities for students in commissionable health-related categories throughout the academic year: the **Junior Commissioned Officer Student Training and Extern Program** (JRCOSTEP) and the **Senior Commissioned Officer Student Training and Extern Program** (SRCOSTEP). Both programs are highly competitive. If you have graduated from an American Council on Pharmaceutical Education (ACPE) accredited program within a year from your call-to-duty date, you may be appointed to the PHS Commissioned Corps for a limited tour of duty that will not exceed one year. Thus, you can become a part of the PHS prior to licensure. In addition, the PHS, in coordination with certain federal agencies, may offer loan repayment and other educational and family support programs.

What pharmacy officers in the PHS Commissioned Corps do

Pharmacists in the Corps care for patients as part of a multidisciplinary healthcare team, conduct biomedical and epidemiological research, and respond to public health emergencies, such as vaccinating patients, assisting hospitals, and coordinating with state and local officials. They may also review, approve, and monitor new drugs or even administer healthcare policy. In addition, there are opportunities to work on organized community disease prevention and treatment programs to improve pharmaceutical care.

Agency assignments

By becoming a part of the PHS, you may choose from a variety of work settings, from working in many agencies, many states, or even overseas. For example, you may begin your career in the Indian Health Service working with Alaska Indians and American Indians, then move to the FDA, then to the CDC, and finally to the NIH. You essentially choose the agency you want to work with. The options for agencies, duties, and locations are endless. The majority of pharmacy officers are assigned to one of the following three agencies:

1. Indian Health Service (IHS) (approximately 47%)
2. Food and Drug Administration (FDA) (approximately 26%)
3. Bureau of Prisons (BoP) (approximately 14%)

As a pharmacist in the PHS, you may be an officer working in any of the following agencies within the HHS. Below is a listing of these agencies and a brief description of what each does:

- **Agency for Healthcare Research and Quality (AHRQ).** The AHRQ supports research designed to improve the outcomes and quality of healthcare, reduce its costs, address patient safety and medical errors, and broaden access to effective services. The research sponsored, conducted, and disseminated by AHRQ provides information that helps people make better decisions about healthcare.

- **Agency for Toxic Substances and Disease Registry (ATSDR).** The ATSDR's mission is to prevent exposure and adverse human health effects and diminished quality of life associated with exposure to hazardous substances from waste sites, unplanned releases, and other sources of pollution present in the environment.

- **Centers for Disease Control and Prevention (CDC).** The CDC's mission is to promote health and quality of life by preventing and controlling disease, injury, and disability. The CDC seeks to accomplish this mission by working with partners throughout the nation and world to monitor health, detect and investigate health problems, conduct research to enhance prevention, develop and advocate sound public health policies, implement prevention strategies, promote healthy behaviors, foster safe and healthful environments, and provide leadership and training.

- **Food and Drug Administration (FDA).** The FDA, one of our nation's oldest consumer protection agencies, ensures the safety of foods and cosmetics, and the safety and efficacy of pharmaceuticals, biological products, and medical devices.

- **Health Resources and Services Administration (HRSA).** The HRSA directs national health programs that improve the nation's health by ensuring equitable access to comprehensive, quality healthcare for all. It works to improve and extend life for people living with HIV/AIDS, provide primary healthcare to medically underserved people, serve women and children through state programs, and train a health workforce that is both diverse and motivated to work in underserved communities.

- **Indian Health Service (IHS).** The IHS is the principal federal healthcare advocate and provider for American Indians and Alaska Natives, who belong to more than 550 federally recognized tribes in 35 States. It provides comprehensive healthcare services, including preventive, curative, rehabilitative, and environmental.

- **National Institutes of Health (NIH).** The NIH with its 27 separate components, mainly Institutes and Centers, is one of the world's foremost medical research centers, and the federal focal point for medical research in the United States. Its mission is to uncover new knowledge that will lead to better health for everyone by conducting research in its own laboratories; supporting the research of nonfederal scientists in universities, hospitals, and research institutions throughout the country and abroad; helping in the training of research investigators; and fostering communication of medical information.

- **Substance Abuse and Mental Health Services Administration (SAMHSA).**
  The SAMHSA works to improve the quality and availability of prevention,
  treatment, and rehabilitative services in order to reduce illness, death, disability, and cost to society resulting from substance abuse and mental illnesses.
- **Office of Public Health and Science (OPHS).** The OPHS is under the direction of the Assistant Secretary for Health, who serves as the senior advisor
  on public health and science issues to the secretary of the HHS. The office
  serves as the focal point of leadership and coordination across the department in public health and science; provides direction to program offices
  within the OPHS; and provides advice and counsel on public health and
  science issues to the secretary.
- **Program Support Center (PSC).** The PSC is a service-for-fee organization
  that utilizes a pioneering business enterprise approach to provide government support services throughout the HHS, as well as other departments
  and federal agencies.

As a PHS Commissioned Officer, you may also be assigned to non-PHS agencies/
programs such as the following:

- U.S. Agency for International Development (USAID)
- Federal Bureau of Prisons (BoP)
- District of Columbia Commission on Mental Health Services (CMHS)
  (formerly St. Elizabeth's Hospital)
- Environmental Protection Agency (EPA)
- Centers for Medicare and Medicaid Services (CMS)
- U.S. Citizenship and Immigration Services (USCIS) (formerly the
  Immigration and Naturalization Service [INS])
- National Oceanic and Atmospheric Administration (NOAA)
- National Park Service (NPS)
- U.S. Coast Guard (USCG)
- U.S. Marshals Service (USMS)
- U.S. Department of Agriculture (USDA)

For more information about pharmacy careers in the PHS, visit the U.S. Public
Health Service website at http://commcorps.shs.net.

OTHER SPECIALIZED FIELDS IN PHARMACY

There are many nontraditional career paths available to pharmacists in such areas as the insurance industry, regulatory agencies, or pharmacy association management. These positions have little patient or medication-use contact. Instead, they often involve new responsibilities and challenges, such as representing pharmacy to other healthcare professionals, the government, and consumer organizations. This challenge, however, is also an opportunity to affect the direction and practice of pharmacy. Pharmacists in these areas generally provide technical expertise on pharmacy practice, using their experience and background to explain the practice of pharmacy to people with limited knowledge of pharmacy and other healthcare areas. Nearly every state has an active pharmaceutical association that employs a full-time executive officer, usually a graduate of a college of pharmacy. In addition, national professional associations are also guided by pharmacists with an interest and special talent in organizational work.

BEYOND THE TYPICAL PHARMACIST ROLE

Still, there are pharmacists who are engaged in a variety of positions, such as in advertising, packaging, technical writing, magazine editing, medical and scientific publishing, and science reporting. There are pharmacists with legal training serving as patent lawyers or as experts in pharmaceutical law. There are pharmacists in America's space laboratories at the National Aeronautics and Space Administration and aboard ships such as the S.S. Hope; others direct large manufacturing firms or specialize in medicinal plant cultivation.

By now, it should be clear that the diversity of pharmacy is one of its chief strengths. The opportunities this profession has to offer are limitless. In the United States, more than 175,000 pharmacists practice in community or hospital pharmacies or long-term and ambulatory care facilities. The remainder follows one or another of the special fields you have just reviewed. As we've stated over and over again, the prospects for immediate employment and for long-term career growth have never been better. The opportunity for success in any of these fields is wide open to anyone with ability, education, and imagination, and definitely a passion to advance the profession of pharmacy.

PART FIVE

Financing Your Degree

CHAPTER 17

Figuring Out Costs

A pharmacy school education is expensive—the total cost can exceed $100,000 depending on the type of institution (public versus private) in which you plan to enroll. However, although the costs are quite hefty, don't despair. If you can demonstrate the determination it takes to make it past the hurdles of being admitted to pharmacy school, financing your education does not have to stand in your way. Just remember that every dollar you spend on your education is a dollar well invested. The returns in direct salary benefits and in other less tangible gains will far exceed your initial investment.

With proper financial planning, it is possible today for nearly every student who meets the necessary academic and personal qualifications to get as much education as they desire and attend the pharmacy school of their choice without worrying about the costs. While the cost may be substantial, it should not deter you, because most institutions offer various mechanisms of financial assistance, making the program accessible to all students, regardless of economic status. The first step in charting a financial path is to know what all of the real costs are. Only then, can you develop a strategy for meeting them, and figure out the costs of your pharmacy education.

TUITION AND FEES

The most natural place to start assessing pharmacy school costs is by looking at tuition and fees. Tuition and fees vary widely from region to region and between public and private institutions. For example, at the public University of Washington School of Pharmacy, annual tuition and fees for in-state residents were $13,454 in 2007–2008. However, at the University of Kentucky College of Pharmacy, also public, tuition and fees for in-state residents were $9,688. For private schools, tuition and fees were as varied as $22,280 annually at Samford University or $35,764 at University of Southern California.

PUBLIC SCHOOLS AND RESIDENCY

Public colleges are almost always less expensive if you are a resident of the state they are located in, because the costs are partially subsidized by state tax revenue. However, attractive low rates for residents may mean that admissions standards are more competitive. If you are a nonresident of the state, very often the added tuition will make your bill look much like that of most private schools. Out-of-state pharmacy students at the University of Washington School of Pharmacy, for example, pay $26,098 in tuition and fees. Out-of-state students at the University of Kentucky College of Pharmacy pay $17,635 annually.

Residency Requirements

While residency requirements vary from state to state, you may be able to gain residency status by living in the state for a year preceding your attendance at the school. If you're planning to attend as a resident of a public institution outside your current state, make sure you check the residency requirements carefully. The time it takes to establish residency varies tremendously from state to state. Check with the staff of the pharmacy school itself for specifics regarding required documentation for establishing residency.

THE BUDGET

Tuition and fees are not the only considerations when figuring out the cost of your pharmacy school education. In assessing total costs, you need to consider the total budget and how much financial aid (scholarship, grant money, etc.) you will receive.

The school's financial aid office estimates the total budget to include all of the standard required costs associated with spending an academic year at the pharmacy school. In addition to tuition and fees, the standard student budget may include the following expenses:

- Books and supplies
- Room and board—living expenses
- Transportation—commuting and parking permits; use of public transportation
- Computer (laptop)
- Miscellaneous personal expenses

Budgets, like expenses, vary depending on your year in school. When financial aid administrators develop the budget, they try to create one that is modest enough to prevent students from over borrowing, and yet adequate enough to recognize realistic costs. Keep in mind that the indirect components of the budget (i.e., living costs, transportation, personal expenses) are average costs based on the specific locale of the school and the specific expenses of the students at that particular school. Whether you apply for aid or not, you can use these average costs to work out a budget from which you can estimate your monthly projected expenses.

What's Not in the Budget

Although the budget is created by each school's financial aid office, it is also governed by federal regulations. The following are a number of items that the government does not allow a school to include:

- **Family expense.** The budget can include only costs for the student, not for the student's spouse/partner or children (although it can include childcare expenses).

- **Optional equipment.** The budget cannot include equipment costs unless the equipment is required for all pharmacy students in the school or for a specific program within the school.
- **Car purchase.** The budget cannot be adjusted for the purchase of a car, even though a car may be required at some point in the program in order for you to travel to clerkships.
- **Relocation.** If you will be attending a pharmacy school that requires you to move, you will have relocation expenses. Expenses that are incurred before your actual enrollment cannot be considered as educational expenses for the purpose of creating a financial aid budget. Thus, your moving costs will be entirely your responsibility. While moving across the country can add thousands of dollars to your first-year expenses, these costs cannot be covered by financial aid.
- **Debt.** Consumer debt is often the most expensive debt around, especially from credit cards. Many students find that they have lingering balances on credit cards from their prepharmacy school lives. If at all possible, pay off what you can before you start pharmacy school.

COMPARING PHARMACY SCHOOL COSTS

Once you understand the basics of what costs are involved in pharmacy school, you can start to make comparisons between what you will actually have to pay to attend different institutions. Try to calculate what you may be allowed for monthly living and other nondirect costs at the pharmacy schools you're considering. Subtract tuition, fees, books, and supplies from the total and divide by the number of months in the academic year. This figure can help you estimate what the financial aid office may determine to be a modest monthly allowance for living while attending the school.

Factor in the Future

"Sure I left pharmacy school with a large school loan to pay, but once I was licensed, the salary made that debt manageable. I live in a rural area and work for a chain drug store."

–Ron, graduate of University of Washington

CALCULATING AID

Once you've figured out your costs, the next step is to determine how much funding a school may provide in scholarship and grant aid. The real issue is not the actual cost, but how much you are going to have to pay. Although private pharmacy schools can seem prohibitive because of hefty tuition charges, some private institutions have endowed awards in the form of grants, scholarships, and low-interest loans. These awards offset their higher costs. Find out from the pharmacy school the percentage of their students that receive some sort of financial assistance, as well as the maximum amount of grant and scholarship funding available from their institution. The more you know, the better able you will be to determine what types of aid are available to you, your eligibility for various programs, and how to approach the financial aid process as a whole.

In chapters 18, 19, and 20, we'll detail the financial aid process as a whole, discuss eligibility for various programs, and explain the best way to apply for each.

CHAPTER 18

Applying for Financial Aid

Financial aid application procedures vary from school to school. It is therefore very important that you contact the institution directly for specifics on the general application requirements and deadlines. The financial aid office offers access to a combination of loans and scholarships that can help you fulfill your financial obligations as long as you apply for assistance and meet the deadline in completing all the required forms.

APPLICATION MATERIALS

Financial aid information is generally provided in the admissions application package so get the admissions materials and read them thoroughly. Pay close attention to financial aid deadlines. Depending on the school, the admissions application deadline can be earlier or later than the financial aid application deadline. In addition, sometimes there are multiple financial aid deadlines: the first one for students interested in scholarship and fellowship assistance, and the later deadline for those who are only interested in federal loans.

FAFSA Form

The most common financial aid application form is the Free Application for Federal Student Aid (FAFSA) form, which is always required to request any federal financial aid. This form is used for "need analysis," the calculation of what you should be able to contribute toward the cost of your education. The detailed financial information you provide on the FAFSA form is then run through a federal formula to arrive at a contribution figure. You can apply for federal financial aid using the FAFSA form on the Web. To do so, go to the U.S. Department of Education website at www.fafsa .ed.gov and follow the step-by-step directions. Although you can still complete a paper FAFSA form, the online process is far more efficient and less time consuming. Remember to apply early because funds may be depleted prior to the deadline dates.

Deadlines

It is important to note the type of deadline you are up against. Be sure to check with the school about their definition of an application deadline, whether it is the *receipt date and time* or the *process date and time* of the application. Although the FAFSA form is the federal application for financial aid, it can also be used to apply for aid from other sources, such as your state or school. The deadlines for your state or school may be different from the federal deadlines because schools have their own deadlines and applications for awarding financial aid. Always check with the school's financial aid office for the most updated information.

SUPPLEMENTAL FINANCIAL AID FORMS

Many pharmacy schools want to know more about you and your family's financial situation in addition to the information you report on the FAFSA form. They usually require that you complete a supplemental application form in addition to the FAFSA in determining your eligibility for the institution's own money. These required forms may include the following:

- Separate school financial aid application
- Parent information statement
- IRS 1040 forms for both the student and parents for the previous year
- Scholarship and outside award documentation

Because some financial aid application deadlines are earlier than April 15, you may not have completed your federal tax forms before the deadline. Most schools recommend that you estimate the numbers and then correct them once you file your taxes. Read the school's financial aid application or check with its financial aid office to find out its policy on estimating tax figures. It is better to estimate a number than to miss a deadline while you're trying to verify it. Just remember to submit the actual figure to the financial aid officer after you have completed your tax forms.

The Student Aid Report (SAR)

The information you provided on your FAFSA form will be used to determine how much you will be expected to contribute toward your educational expenses for the upcoming school year. After submitting the FAFSA, you will receive a Student Aid Report (SAR) from the federal processor by email. Read the SAR carefully! Be sure to check that all potential pharmacy schools of your choice are included in the school list section so that they will receive your application information. You must follow SAR instructions for submitting a school change or addition. If data you reported is incorrect or failed any of the database matches, you must follow the instructions given to correct or resolve matters. The most common causes of database mismatches are incorrect names, birth dates, and citizenship status. If all the information is accurate, you have completed this part of the application process.

CALCULATING YOUR NEED

Your financial need or eligibility is based on the evaluation of the information from the FAFSA, your (and your parents) IRS 1040 tax forms, and any other documentation requested. Factors specifically considered are income, assets, family size, age of the primary wage earner, and number of dependent children in the family who are attending postsecondary institutions. Financial aid eligibility is based on both the student's need and the availability of funds. The financial need is determined using the following formula:

Cost of Attendance – Family Contribution = Financial Need

The cost of attendance is determined by the school and consists of tuition and fees, living expenses, books and supplies, transportation, and personal expenses. The family contribution reflects an estimate of the family's ability to meet the cost of attendance. The formula used to determine the family contribution is based on the nationally accepted formula known as Federal Methodology (FM).

Federal Methodology (FM)

A need analysis method developed by Congress is used to calculate the Family Contribution (FC). The FM determines eligibility for federal student aid programs.

The FAFSA form that you file gives enough information to the federal processor to run your figures through this formula and produce an Expected Family Contribution (EFC). The federal processor is a selected firm under the U.S. government contract who uses the methodology approved by Congress to calculate your contributions.

Dependent or Independent?

For programs that receive funding through the U.S. Department of Education, pharmacy students are considered independent. This means that your parents' financial information is not used to determine your EFC and not used to determine your need for federal programs offered by the U.S. Department of Education. Examples of programs for which you are automatically considered independent include Federal Stafford Loans, Federal Perkins Loans, or Federal Work-Study. These programs are available to students regardless of their family's background.

However, for some programs funded by the U.S. Department of Health and Human Services and many institutional funds, students are considered dependent. This means that your parents' income and asset information will be required to determine your EFC and need for those programs. In fact, many pharmacy schools award their institutional grants, scholarships, and low-interest loan funds based on both student and parent financial information. Therefore, these schools request that all students provide parental information to be considered for all available funds. Independent students are also to submit their parents' information to be considered for the Scholarship for Disadvantaged Students, Loan for Disadvantaged Students, and the Health Professions Student Loan.

Independence

Programs for which you are automatically considered independent:

- Federal Stafford Loans
- William T. Ford Direct Loans
- Federal Perkins Loans
- Federal Work-Study

Family Affairs

Federal health professions programs for which you will be considered dependent:

- Scholarships for Disadvantaged Students (SDS)
- Loans for Disadvantaged Students (LDS)
- Primary Care Loans (PCL)

Thus, many schools consider the parents' financial circumstances even when students are financially independent. Remember, priority for campus-based funds is given to students who are found to be most needy and have submitted the required documents by the deadlines!

DETERMINING THE EXPECTED FAMILY CONTRIBUTION

The EFC is based on the income and asset information reported on the FAFSA. In assessing the EFC for an independent student, the following components are considered and used in the Federal Methodology:

- Total family income from the previous year (base year income)
- Net value of any assets (excluding home equity)
- Taxes paid (federal, state, local)
- Asset protection allowance. This allowance provides protection of assets depending on your age. A portion of your assets will not be considered in the calculation because they are protected for purposes other than education, such as emergencies or retirement. The older you are, the more your assets are protected.
- Number of family members
- Social Security tax allowance. The calculation of Social Security tax is based on existing federal rates applied to income earned from work and may never be less than zero.
- Income protection allowance. This allowance provides for basic living expenses not included in the standard student expense budget. It will vary according to the number of family members and the number in college at least half-time.

FEDERAL METHODOLOGY

The FM determines an applicant's eligibility for most federal financial aid programs. The formula takes the income that is received by the members of the student's household, subtracts the taxes paid and the cost of maintaining the members of the family other than the student, adds in a portion of the assets, and then takes a percentage of the result to produce a family contribution. Although this formula may not take into account all aspects of an individual student's situation, it produces generally comparable data on all students applying for financial aid.

GRADUATE CLASSIFICATION

A student's classification as an undergraduate or a graduate student may qualify them for additional funding. Students with three or more years of college work or more than 90 semester units (or 135 quarter units) are considered to be graduate students for federal, state, and university financial aid funding. First-year pharmacy students who matriculate *without* a bachelor's degree and with transferable units (as determined by the institution) that total *fewer* than 135 quarter or 90 semester units can apply for additional need-based grants that are designed for undergraduates. For example, such undergraduate students with exceptional financial need would qualify for the Federal Pell Grants and Federal Supplemental Educational Opportunity Grants. If you do not hold a bachelor's degree by the time you start pharmacy school and are uncertain of your classification as either an undergraduate or graduate student, you should contact the pharmacy school's financial aid office for counseling to determine whether you qualify for additional need-based funding.

WHAT TO EXPECT NEXT

My Heart Was Set

A top pharmacy school and a lesser-known school may accept you. What do you do? Many applicants have their hearts set on going to top-flight schools, but accept offers from others that are more generous with their aid packages. Be prepared to weigh all offers based on many factors—including cost.

Once your financial aid application is complete, the financial aid office will often wait for the admissions decision before they review your application and determine your eligibility. When the financial aid office finds out that you have been accepted, they will make an offer of financial aid. This offer is called a financial aid package or an official financial aid offer letter.

Now you need to review the financial aid packages and decide where you'll attend pharmacy school. Your choice may not be the school that offered you the largest scholarship. You need to weigh the merits of the financial aid package against the desirability of the school itself.

HOW AID IS AWARDED

Financial aid awards are made each year based on the total assessed need of the applicants and the amount of funds available. Awards vary year-to-year depending on allocations received from federal, state, and university funding sources. Remember that financial aid is awarded on a priority basis; thus, applications completed by the stated deadlines are processed and awarded first. Applications completed after the deadline risk losing available funding sources because they are given out on a first-come, first-served basis.

Financial need represents the total amount of assistance for which you are eligible. Your financial aid package can include any combination of need-based aid, fellowships, assistantships, scholarships, grants, or federal and private loans. These awards may not exceed the estimated federal contribution calculated from the financial aid need analysis formula. You should carefully evaluate your financial aid package and determine the following:

- What is your contribution expected to be?
- How much will you be expected to borrow?
- What kinds of loans are offered? What are the rates and repayment terms?

These questions should be answered before you make your admissions decision.

CHAPTER 19

Finding Free Money

It is every student's dream to get "free money"—money you don't have to pay back—to pay for their pharmacy school education. Free money can come from a variety of sources, including federal and state governments, schools themselves, and private donors.

FEDERAL FUNDS

Both the U.S. Department of Education and the Department of Health and Human Services allocate funds yearly for the education of health professionals such as pharmacists. For some programs, participating institutions also contribute money. Eligibility for federal programs is based on financial need as well as other factors.

Scholarships for Disadvantaged Students (SDS)

This scholarship is awarded to full-time, financially needy students from disadvantaged backgrounds enrolled in health professions programs. For more information on the definitions of "financial need" and "disadvantaged" for this specific program, contact the financial aid office. Scholarships may not exceed the cost of attendance. That is, tuition, reasonable educational expenses, and reasonable living expenses.

STATE FUNDS

Some states have grant programs available to pharmacy students that are often based on financial need as well as other criteria, such as state residency. You should contact the financial aid office to determine if such programs exist in your state.

INSTITUTIONAL FUNDS

Some pharmacy schools will have a pool of funding they call institutional grants or scholarships. While some of this funding is reserved for awards made strictly on the basis of merit, for the most part this is the money schools direct toward students based on need in order to equalize grant and loan awards. Other than the small pot administered through the Department of Health and Human Services that is designated for students with need from disadvantaged backgrounds, these are the only "free money" types of aid the institution has discretion in awarding. You can bet the aid office goes through some pretty amazing calculations to determine who receives these funds. Parental information is usually required to determine eligibility for institutional grants and scholarships, and it is evaluated carefully before awards are made from these funds.

Most pharmacy schools also have scholarships that are awarded from endowed funds donated by an individual or organization and named for an individual. Pharmacy colleges also administer student financial assistance funds provided by local or state pharmaceutical associations and their auxiliaries, community and independent pharmacies, practicing pharmacists, drug manufacturers and wholesalers, memorial funds and foundations, alumni associations, local chapters of pharmaceutical organizations and fraternities, as well as general university funds allocated for this purpose. These are all considered free dollars. They typically are awarded based on the donor's eligibility criteria and can require some form of communication with the donor. The aid office will often let you know if any of these programs are appropriate for you.

Awards can range from hundreds to thousands of dollars. Each dollar you receive as a grant or scholarship from these sources could equal at least two dollars you won't have to repay to a loan program.

PHARMACY EDUCATION FINANCIAL PROGRAMS DATABASE

The Pharmacy Education Financial Programs (PEFP) document is an online financial aid database. It contains scholarship, loan, grant, and award information for current professional and graduate pharmacy students. The PEFP is a valuable resource for pharmacy students seeking additional financial support and professional recognition. The PEFP is compiled annually by the 10-member organizations of the Career Information Clearinghouse (CIC), a collection of national pharmacy-related organizations that collaborate on the development of materials designed to recruit and assist prospective and professional pharmacy students. CIC members include:

- American Association of Colleges of Pharmacy
- American College of Apothecaries
- American Society of Consultant Pharmacists
- American Society of Health-System Pharmacists
- Academy of Managed Care Pharmacy
- Healthcare Distribution Management Association
- National Association of Chain Drug Stores
- National Community Pharmacists Association
- Pharmaceutical Research and Manufacturers of America
- The American Pharmacists Association

The PEFP database is hosted on the National Association of Chain Drug Stores website at www.nacds.org/wmspage.cfm?parm1=2912.

ADDITIONAL SCHOLARSHIP SEARCH DATABASES

You are encouraged to investigate sources of financial assistance beyond what is offered by the federal and state governments and their schools. Many of these awards are based on a wide variety of qualifications including financial need, academic achievement, religious affiliation, ethnicity, special interests, or pharmacy practice specialty.

The Internet can provide a wealth of information on these resources. However, keep in mind that these free scholarship searches will be useful only if the database is up-to-date. More importantly, you still have to apply for the funds and will probably need to complete a detailed application. Before you actually spend the time applying, check to see that the award amount is commensurate with the time you have to put into applying. The following is a sample list of free searchable databases:

- FastWEB. This is an extremely popular database with more than 600,000 private sector scholarships, fellowships, grants, and loans. *(www.fastweb.com)*

- The SmartStudent Guide to Financial Aid. This is an extremely comprehensive guide to all student financial aid information and free scholarship, grant, and fellowship search databases. *(www.finaid.org)*

- NextStudent Scholarship Search Engine. This is one of the oldest scholarship databases and contains over 800,000 scholarships based on many different qualifications and a broad range of criteria, such as academic achievements, community services, family heritage, and special talents or aptitude. *(www.nextstudent.com)*

CHAPTER 20

Borrowing the Money

Student loans are an important source of support for pharmacy students. Pharmacy schools expect the majority of students with financial need will borrow at least part of their educational costs. You should research loan possibilities early in the financial aid application process. It can take weeks from the date you applied to receive the loan proceeds, so planning is essential. Also, note that the rules and regulations for borrowing through each of these programs differ.

FEDERAL LOAN PROGRAMS

The U.S. Department of Education disburses the following two federal loan programs that are available to pharmacy students and generally considered the core loan programs featuring a low interest rate, low fees, and defined deferment provisions:

1. *Federal Stafford Student Loan Program* (part of the Federal Family Education Loan Program, FFEL), also referred to as FFEL Stafford Loans
2. *William D. Ford Federal Direct Student Loan Program*, also referred to as Ford Federal Direct Loans

Most terms and conditions of these two loans are similar, including eligibility criteria, interest rates, grace period, deferment, and cancellation provisions.

The major differences between the two are the source of the loan funds, some aspects of the application process, and the available repayment plans. Under the Direct Loan Program, funds are loaned to the student directly by the U.S. government. When a school does not participate in the Direct Loan Program, funds are loaned to the student from a private lender (such as a bank, credit union, or other lender that participates in the FFEL Stafford Loan Program). Most pharmacy institutions participate in the FFEL Stafford Program, but only some participate in the Ford Direct Programs. The school you attend will determine which of these two loans you can apply for. Depending on when you first borrow, there's a grace period of six or nine months before you'll have to start repayment.

Interest Rates

FFEL Stafford and Ford Direct Loans are either *subsidized* or *unsubsidized*. A borrower can receive a subsidized loan and an unsubsidized loan for the same enrollment period. The interest rate on these loans may not exceed 8.25 percent.

More Benefits of Research

"The National Institutes of Health has a wonderful program to pay school loan debt if one commits to an academic career based in research. This program really helped me after I became an assistant professor."

–Shannon, graduate of University of California–San Francisco

A *subsidized* loan is awarded on the basis of financial need. The borrower will not be charged any interest before repayment begins or during authorized periods of deferment. The federal government "subsidizes" the interest during these periods.

An *unsubsidized* loan is not awarded on the basis of need. The borrower will be charged interest from the time the loan is disbursed until it is paid in full. You are responsible for the interest while you're in school, but most lenders will allow you to defer the interest, and not pay it until you leave school. However, if interest is allowed to accumulate, it will be capitalized; that is, the interest will be added to the principal amount of the loan and additional interest will be based upon the higher amount, thereby, increasing the total amount the borrower will have to repay.

Borrowing Limits

Pharmacy students may borrow up to their demonstrated need with a maximum of $8,500 per year in the Federal Subsidized Stafford Loan Program. The Federal Unsubsidized Stafford Loan Program allows an eligible student to borrow up to $24,500 per year, minus any Subsidized Stafford Loan approved. The annual total Stafford limit for pharmacy is $33,000. The borrowing limits are the same for the Ford Direct Loans.

Deferments

Under certain circumstances you may be able to defer, or postpone, the payments of your federal loans. Deferments are not automatic, rather you must apply for them.

Forbearance

You can request forbearance in situations that are not covered by normal deferments. Forbearance means the lender agrees to grant you a temporary suspension of payments, reduced payments, or an extension of the time for your payments.

Repayment

For the FFEL Federal Stafford Loan Program, the amount of your monthly payment will depend on the total amount you borrowed, the number of months in the repayment schedule, the type of repayment schedule, and whether you elected to pay interest on the unsubsidized portion of the loan while in school. A typical repayment period is usually 10 years. Lenders are required to offer the option of standard, graduated, or income-sensitive repayment to new borrowers.

> **Promissory Notes**
>
> Terms of repayment are explained in your promissory note. Be sure that you understand them. Keep the promissory note; it's your contract with the lender.

If you don't meet the repayment terms of the loan, you'll go into default and the entire balance of the loan becomes due. Check with your lender to explore repayment plan options. Lenders are trying to make it possible for you to stay in good standing with your repayments, and they're willing to work with you to help you manage your debt.

For the Ford Direct Loan Program, most of the conditions of repayment are the same as the Stafford Loan Program except that students in the Direct Loan Program have three repayment options in addition to the standard:

1. *Option 1: Extended repayment.*

   This is similar to the standard repayment plan but allows you to repay a fixed amount over a period longer than 10 years.

2. *Option 2: Income contingent repayment.*

   You pay a percentage of your salary no matter how much you have borrowed. If you have a high debt, this option could require many more years of repayment than the standard 10 years. The drawback to this option is that the longer you stay in repayment, the more interest you pay on the loan. If your payment does not cover current interest due, unpaid interest will be capitalized and thus increase the amount of principal you owe.

Generous Employers

"I took out $120,000 worth of school loans to pay for pharmacy school, but once I became a Commissioned Officer in the U.S. Public Health Service and agreed to serve in the Indian Health Service, they started paying off my school loans."

—Pat, pharmacist

---

3. *Option 3: Graduated repayment.*

   This allows you to opt for lower payments at the beginning of the repayment cycle when your salary is lower. The payments automatically increase as the years progress. The repayment term may be extended beyond 10 years, but the payments are more manageable in the beginning when you probably have a lower salary.

PLUS LOANS

In addition, the FFEL Federal Stafford Student Loan Program and the Ford Direct Loan Program also offer PLUS Loans for parents of dependent students. Most of the benefits to parent borrowers are identical in the two programs. PLUS loans enable parents with good credit histories to borrow to pay the educational expenses of each child who is a dependent undergraduate student enrolled at least half-time.

FEDERAL PERKINS STUDENT LOAN

Administered by pharmacy institutions, the Federal Perkins Loan Program is made possible through a combination of resources: an annual allocation from the U.S. Department of Education, a contribution from the participating educational institution, and repayments by previous borrowers. This subsidized loan, which has a 5 percent interest rate, is available to eligible undergraduate and graduate students, with priority going to students who have exceptional need. Loan limits are $4,000 per year or $20,000 cumulative for undergraduate students, and $6,000 per year or $40,000 cumulative for graduate students (including loans received as undergraduates). However, many schools lack the funds to allocate this much to any one student. Interest and repayment begin nine months after the borrower completes his or her course of study.

HEALTH PROFESSIONS STUDENT LOANS

Health Professions Student Loans provide long-term, low-interest loans to full-time financially needy students pursuing a degree in the health professions such as pharmacy. Through the U.S. Department of Health and Human Services, the funds are made available to schools for the establishment of revolving student loan funds. Students apply at the student aid office of the school of their choice for assistance in applying for the loan. The program provides 5 percent loans to pharmacy students. Parents' financial information must be analyzed annually, regardless of the student's age or dependency status, to determine whether a contribution to the cost of education is expected. Repayment and interest begin one year after the student ceases full-time studies or obtains the first professional degree. The maximum that can be borrowed for a nine-month period of attendance varies by institution (in general, from $2,000 to $6,500 per year).

LOANS FOR DISADVANTAGED STUDENTS

Loans for Disadvantaged Students (LDS) funds are available to pharmacy students from disadvantaged backgrounds. Disadvantaged background means that a student comes from an unusually low family income or from an environment that has inhibited him or her from obtaining the knowledge, skills, and abilities required to enroll in and graduate from a health professions program. The LDS program provides

5 percent loans. Parents' financial information must be analyzed annually, regardless of the student's age or dependency status, to determine whether a contribution to the cost of education is expected. Repayment and interest begin one year after the student ceases full-time studies or obtains the first professional degree. The maximum that can be borrowed for a nine-month period of attendance varies by institution, but annual awards usually may not exceed tuition plus $2,500.

PRIVATE LOANS

Many student loan programs are made available through pharmacy organizations and community pharmacy chains. For example, the National Community Pharmacists Association (NCPA) Foundation has assisted hundreds of pharmacy students in financing their education by providing more than $5.5 million in low-interest-rate loans. Applicants must be student members of the NCPA and be enrolled in an accredited U.S. school or college of pharmacy. Applicants may apply for a maximum loan amount of $2,500 per semester, depending on tuition and book fees, with a $5,000 maximum per year and a total loan maximum of $17,500. The interest rate is prime plus 0.5 percent, which accrues annually beginning 90 days after graduation. The National Association of Chain Drug Stores (NACDS) Foundation offers pharmacy students the *Loan to Learn* program, which provides information and access to education loans that are based on borrower credit and income, unlike federal loans that are based solely on financial need. The loans may provide funds for comprehensive education costs including tuition and fees, room and board, books and supplies, study abroad, and computers. The Rite Aid-Wells Fargo Concern Loan Program is a pharmacy student loan provided by Wells Fargo through Rite Aid Corporation. Applicants must be interns at Rite Aid and enrolled in a pharmacy program. Up to $25,000 per year may be awarded to successful applicants. Further information on numerous pharmacy specialty private loans can be searched on the PEFP database.

LOAN REPAYMENT PROGRAMS (LRP)

There are several loan programs under which you promise to work in exchange for reduced levels of debt. While they require time commitment, they can reduce the size of your educational debt tremendously. Many states have initiated loan repayment (or forgiveness) programs for pharmacists who agree to practice in high-need or rural areas. Below are a couple of examples of different types of LRP. Indian Health

Service (IHS) Loan Repayment Program Participants are required to practice clinical pharmacy by providing direct patient care at an IHS or other Indian health program priority site for two continuous years. In return, the LRP will repay up to $20,000 per year for each year of service. National Institutes of Health (NIH) Loan Repayment Program This LRP is designed to attract health professionals to careers in clinical, pediatric, health disparities, or contraception and infertility research. In exchange for a two-year commitment to your research career, NIH will repay up to $35,000 per year of your qualified educational debt.

FEDERAL LOAN CONSOLIDATION

Federal Loan Consolidation allows students with substantial debt to combine several federal loans into one larger loan with a longer repayment schedule. The new loan has an interest rate based on the weighted average of the rates of the consolidated loans and may not exceed 8.25 percent. Stafford Loans, Federal Insured Student Loans (FISLs), Federal Perkins Loans, PLUS loans to students, parent PLUS loans made after 1986, Health Professions Student Loans, Health Education Assistance Loans, and Nursing Student Loan Program loans may be consolidated only by lenders that have an agreement with the Department or a guaranty agency for that purpose.

To qualify for federal loan consolidation, you must be in the grace period or in repayment status on all loans being consolidated; if in default, you must have made satisfactory arrangements to repay the defaulted loan. To consolidate a defaulted loan, you must make three consecutive reasonable and affordable monthly payments. A borrower in default can qualify for a Federal Consolidation Loan without having to make three required payments if the borrower agrees to repay the loan under the income-sensitive repayment plan.

Furthermore, a borrower in default must not have another consolidation loan application pending; must agree to notify the loan holder of any address changes; and must certify that the lender holds the borrower's outstanding loan that is being consolidated, or that the borrower has unsuccessfully sought a loan from the holders of the outstanding loans, and was unable to secure a consolidation loan from the holder.

If you are unable to obtain a Federal Consolidation Loan from a lender eligible to make such loans, you may apply through the U.S. Department of Education for a Federal Direct Consolidation Loan. You must certify that you have been unable to obtain a Federal Consolidation Loan or a Federal Consolidation Loan from an eligible lender with income-sensitive repayment terms acceptable to the borrower.

You have the option of consolidating all eligible loans or only some of your loans. No fees are charged to participate in this program.

If you consolidate your loans, you have the option of choosing the most appropriate repayment plan for you and your circumstances. These options include level repayment, graduated repayment, or income-sensitive repayment.

DEBT MANAGEMENT

Borrowing money means taking on a serious obligation to repay with interest in the future. You should carefully assess the total educational indebtedness and your ability to repay these debts after graduation. When possible, repay your loans early so that you will have less interest to pay and will make the funds available to others. There is no penalty for early repayment. In many cases, there will be no interest if the loan is repaid before the grace period expires.

Student loans generally have a "grace period" that starts when borrowers graduate or withdraw from school and lasts six months to one year. Repayment on student loans begins at the end of the grace period. However, if you've changed schools or returned to school, you can generally defer repayment of your student loans. A continuance of in-school status occurs when individuals have not yet used the grace period and are transitioning from an undergraduate to a graduate program. During deferment or continuance of in-school status, interest on loans does not accrue and repayment is not required. Loans go into default when the lender expects payment and you fail to make the payments. Therefore, if your projected indebtedness seems unmanageable, you should try to figure out ways to reduce your borrowing.

Use the worksheet on the next page to calculate your monthly repayments after graduation.

WILL MY PAYCHECK COVER MY EXPENSES?

Income

1. My annual salary/wages $_____
2. My spouse/partner's salary/wages   _____
3. Other income (source/amount) (e.g., interest, self-employment, etc.; don't include gifts that may not be available each year)   _____
4. Total annual income (sum of lines 1–3)   _____
5. Monthly income (line 4 divided by 12)   _____

Mandatory Expenses

6. Taxes   _____
7. Monthly mandatory deductions from salary (e.g., health insurance, required pension contribution)   _____
8. My monthly student loan payment (assume $125 per $10,000 of student loans)   _____
9. My spouse/partner's monthly student loan payment   _____
10. My total monthly personal debt payments (credit card and other personal debts; assume minimum payment of 3 percent of total credit card balance)   _____
11. My spouse/partner's total monthly personal debt payments   _____
12. Total of what I have to pay each month (sum of lines 6–11)   _____

Discretionary Monthly Income

13. Total monthly income (line 5)   _____
14. Total monthly mandatory expenses (line 12)   _____
15. Monthly total available for living expenses (line 14 minus line 13)   _____

Living Expenses/Discretionary Expenses

16. Rent/mortgage and maintenance fees   _____
17. Utilities and phone (local and long distance)   _____
18. Groceries and meals away from home (including lunches at work)   _____
19. Clothing, laundry, dry cleaning   _____
20. Medical and dental care, prescriptions   _____
21. Recreation, entertainment (also include newspapers, magazines, TV/cable)   _____
22. Car (payments, parking, gas, insurance, repairs) or mass transit expenses   _____
23. Vacation/travel   _____
24. Dependent or child care   _____
25. Insurance (home, life, medical, dental, renter's)   _____
26. Personal care   _____
27. Gifts, miscellaneous   _____
28. Savings, emergency fund, retirement (emergency fund should equal 3–6 mo. salary; recommended level of savings/retirement investment = 10% of gross monthly income)   _____
29. Total monthly living and discretionary expenses (sum of lines 16–28)   _____
30. Total monthly amount of money remaining and available for savings, investment, improved life style (line 15 minus line 29)   _____
31. Annual amount of money remaining (line 30 times 12)   _____

PART SIX

Resources

Quick Reference
List of Key Resources

Academy of Managed Care Pharmacy (AMCP)

100 N. Pitt Street, Suite 400
Alexandria, VA 22314
Phone: 800-827-2627
Website: www.amcp.org
Listing of the available managed care residencies nationwide.

Accreditation Council for Pharmacy Education (ACPE)

20 N. Clark Street, Suite 2500
Chicago, IL 60602-5109
Phone: (312) 664-3575
Website: www.acpe-accredit.org
Find out the accreditation status of pharmacy schools.

American Association of Colleges of Pharmacy (AACP)

1727 King Street
Alexandria, VA 22314
Phone: (703) 739-2330
Website: www.aacp.org
The AACP is the primary resource for pharmacy school applicants. Get information on the Pharmacy College Admission Test (PCAT), the Pharmacy College Application Service (PharmCAS), the Pharmacy School Admission Requirements (PSAR) guide, as well as other extensive information on attending pharmacy school.

American College of Clinical Pharmacy (ACCP)

13000 W. 87th St. Parkway
Lenexa, KS 66215-4530
Phone: (913) 492-3311
Website: www.accp.com
Listing of available residencies.

American Pharmacists Association (APhA)

2215 Constitution Avenue, NW
Washington, DC 20037
Phone: (202) 628-4410
Website: www.pharmacist.com
Listing of community pharmacy residency programs.

American Society of Health-System Pharmacists (ASHP)

7272 Wisconsin Avenue
Bethesda, MD 20814
Phone: 866-279-0681
Website: www.ashp.org
Listing of available residencies.

The National Association of Boards of Pharmacy (NABP)

1600 Feehanville Drive
Mount Prospect, IL 60056
Phone: (847) 391-4406
Website: www.nabp.net
Information on the pharmacy licensure examinations:
the North American Pharmacist Licensure Examination
(NAPLEX) and the Multistate Pharmacy Jurisprudence
Examination (MPJE).

National Association of Chain Drug Stores (NACDS)

413 N. Lee Street
P.O. Box 1417-D49
Alexandria, VA 22313-1480
Phone: (703) 549-3001
Website: www.nacds.org
Listing of available scholarships, internships,
and residencies.

National Community Pharmacists Association (NCPA)

100 Daingerfield Road
Alexandria, VA 22314
Phone: (703) 683-8200
Website: www.ncpanet.org
For those interested in community pharmacy, this
website provides information on student scholarships,
internships, and the opportunities available to pharma-
cists practicing in a community or independent setting.

Pharmacy College Admission Test (PCAT)

Phone: 800-622-3231
Website: www.pcatweb.info

Pharmacy College Application Service (PharmCAS)

P.O. Box 9109
Watertown, MA 02471
Phone: (617) 612-2050
Website: www.pharmcas.org

PharmD Gateway to NIH

Website: www.nigms.nih.gov/Training/PharmD
This website provides information about National
Institutes of Health (NIH) funding opportunities for
PharmD students, postdoctoral researchers, and faculty
interested in biomedical and behavioral research.

Pharmacy School Statistics

There are over 100 pharmacy institutions in the United States. For the accreditation status of each program, contact the Accreditation Council for Pharmacy Education. The statistics (2006-2007) provided below may vary from year to year. Contact each individual program for the most up to date information.

Albany College of Pharmacy

106 New Scotland Avenue, Albany, NY 12208
Phone: (518) 694-7221 **Fax:** (518) 445-7294
Website: www.acp.edu
General Info: Private school with an acceptance rate of 25% to pharmacy school. **Pharmacy Student Body:** 1,400 **Male/Female Ratio:** 43/57 **Joint Degrees Offered:** PharmD/MBA, PharmD/JD **PCAT:** Not Required **PharmCAS:** Required **Minimum GPA:** 3.2 **Average GPA:** 3.6 **Early Admissions Deadline:** November 1 **Application Deadline:** February 1 **Application Fee:** $100 **In-State Tuition:** $22,050 **Out-of-State Tuition:** $22,050 **Prerequisites:** English (8 semester hours), General Chemistry I and II (8 semester hours), General Biology I and II (8 semester hours), Organic Chemistry I and II (8 semester hours), Statistics I (3 semester hours), Microbiology (4 semester hours), Calculus I (3 semester hours), Liberal Arts Electives (18 semester hours), Other electives (8 semester hours). *Satellite campus at Colchester, VT

Appalachian College of Pharmacy

1060 Dragon Road, Oakwood, VA 24631
Phone: (276) 498-4190
Website: www.acpharm.org
General Info: Private school with an acceptance rate of 33% to pharmacy school. **Pharmacy Student Body:** 195 **Male/Female Ratio:** 49/51

Students per Class: 65 **Joint Degrees Offered:** None **PCAT:** Required **PharmCAS:** Required **Minimum GPA:** 2.50 **Average GPA:** 3.15 **Application Deadline:** March 1 **Application Fee:** $100 **In-State Tuition:** $32,500 **Out-of-State Tuition:** $32,500 **Prerequisites:** Biology w/Lab (8 semester hours), Chemistry w/Lab (8 semester hours), Organic Chemistry w/Lab (8 semester hours), College Physics w/Lab (8 semester hours), Human Anatomy (3 semester hours), Human Physiology (3 semester hours), General Microbiology (3 semester hours), English Composition (6 semester hours), Math (6 semester hours), Public speaking (3 semester hours), Statistics (3 semester hours), Electives (10 semester hours).

Auburn University Harrison School of Pharmacy

2316 Walker Building, Auburn University, AL 36849-5501
Phone: (334) 844-8348 **Fax:** (334) 844-8353
Website: www.pharmacy.auburn.edu
General Info: Private school **Pharmacy Student Body:** 480 **Male/Female Ratio:** 30/70 **Students per Class:** 125 **Joint Degrees Offered:** None **PCAT:** Required **Minimum Score:** 45% **PharmCAS:** Required **Minimum GPA:** 2.5 **Average GPA:** 3.3 **Early Admissions Deadline:** September 1 **Application Deadline:** March 1 **Application Fee:** $50 **In-State Tuition:** $15,384

Out-of-State Tuition: $24,200 Prerequisites: English Composition (6 semester hours), English World Literature (6 semester hours), Calculus (4 semester hours), Biology I w/Lab (4 semester hours), World History I and II (6 semester hours), Chemistry I and II w/Lab (8 semester hours), Biology: anatomy & physiology I and II (8 semester hours), Biology: genomic biology or perspectives in immunology (4 semester hours), Organic Chemistry I and II w/Lab (8 semester hours), Microbiology (4 semester hours), Biochemistry (3 semester hours), Physics (4 semester hours), Fine Arts (3 semester hours), Philosophy: ethics and health sciences (3 semester hours), Social Sciences (6 semester hours), Statistics (3 semester hours).

Belmont University School of Pharmacy

1900 Belmont Blvd., Nashville, TN 37212
Phone: 615-460-6000
Website: www.belmont.edu/pharmacy
General Info: Belmont University is a private school. Pharmacy student body: 150 (inaugural class 2008) Male/Female Ratio: 36/64 Class Size: 75 Joint Degrees Offered: None PCAT required: Yes PharmCAS required: Yes Minimum GPA: 2.7 Average GPA: 3.3 Early admissions: Yes Application deadline: March 1 Application fee: $50 In-State Tuition: $25,440 Out-of-State Tuition: $25,440 Prerequisites: Literature (3 semester hours), English Composition (3 semester hours); Writing Emphasis (3 semester hours), Biology w/ lab (8 semester hours), Physics w/ lab (4 semester hours); General Chemistry w/ lab (8 semester hours), Organic Chemistry w/lab (8 semester hours), Calculus (4 semester hours), Statistics: 3, General or Health Economics (3 semester hours), Public Speaking (3 semester hours), Social science electives (9 semester hours), Electives (6 semester hours)

Butler University College of Pharmacy and Health Sciences

4600 Sunset Avenue, Indianapolis, IN 46208
Phone: (317)940-8100 Fax: (317) 940-8150
Website: www.butler.edu/cophs
General Info: Private School with an acceptance rate of 17.5% to pharmacy school Pharmacy Student Body: 525 Male/Female Ratio: 31/69

Students per Class: 160 Joint Degrees Offered: PharmD/MBA PCAT: Required Minimum Score: 55% PharmCAS: Required Minimum GPA: 3.0 Application Deadline: February 1. Application Fee: $100 In-State Tuition: $26,670 Out-of-State Tuition: $26,670 Prerequisites: General Chemistry (10 semester hours), Organic Chemistry (10 semester hours), Introductory Cell Biology (3 semester hours), Human Anatomy (3 semester hours), Pathogenic Microbiology (3 semester hours), Calculus and Analytical Geometry (5 semester hours), Human Anatomy (3 semester hours).

California Northstate College of Pharmacy

10811 International Drive, Rancho Cordova, CA 95670 Phone: 916-631-8108
Website: www.californiacollegeofpharmacy.org
General Info: CNCP is a private school and it has an acceptance rate of 21.3% to its pharmacy school. Male/Female Ratio: 44/56 Class Size: 80 Joint Degrees Offered: None PCAT required: No PharmCAS required: Yes Minimum GPA: 2.7 Average GPA: 3.22 Early admissions: No; Application deadline: February 1 Application fee: $60 In-State Tuition: $36,400 Out-of-State Tuition: $36,400 Pre-requisites: General Chemistry w/ lab (2 semesters), Organic Chemistry w/lab (2 semesters), General Biology w/lab (2 semesters), Physiology or Anatomy & Physiology (1 semester); Microbiology: 1 semester), Biochemistry or Cell & Molecular Biology (1 semester), Physics with lab (1 semester); Calculus (1 semester); Psychology (1 semester); Macro or micro economics (1 semester), Public speaking (1 semester)

Campbell University School of Pharmacy

P.O. Box 1090, 205 Day Dorm Road, Room 101, Buies Creek, NC 27506
Phone: (910) 893-1690 Fax: (910) 893-1943
Website: www.campbellpharmacy.net
General Info: Private school with an acceptance rate of 7% to pharmacy school Pharmacy Student Body: 450 Male/Female Ratio: 35/65 Student/Faculty Ratio: 9/1 Students per Class: 105 Joint Degrees Offered: PharmD/MBA, PharmD/MSPS, PharmD/MSCR PCAT: Required Minimum Score: 65% PharmCAS: Required Minimum GPA: 2.5 Average GPA: 3.4 Application

Deadline: February 1 **Application Fee:** $25
In-State Tuition: $26,000 **Out-of-State Tuition:**
$26,000 **Prerequisites:** English Composition (6
semester hours), Religion: bible-based course (3
semester hours), Humanities (6 semester hours),
Social Sciences (6 semester hours), Economics/
Accounting (3 semester hours), Physical Education
(2 semester hours), Calculus (3 semester hours),
Physics (4 semester hours), General Chemistry (8
semester hours), Organic Chemistry (8 semester
hours), Biological Sciences (8 semester hours),
Electives (12 semester hours).

Chicago State University College of Pharmacy

9501 S. King Drive, 206 Douglas Hall, Chicago, IL
60628-1598
Phone: (773) 821-2000 **Website:** www.csu.edu/
collegeofpharmacy/index.htm
General Info: Public school. **Pharmacy Student
Body:** Expects to admit 78 students into its
inaugural class upon matriculation in 2008.
Joint Degrees Offered: None **PCAT:** Required
PharmCAS: Not required **Minimum GPA:** 2.5
Average GPA: TBD **Application Deadline:** TBD
Application Fee: TBD **In-State Tuition:** $17,500
Out-of-State Tuition: $26,250 **Prerequisites:**
English Composition (6 semester hours), Biology
(8 semester hours), Anatomy: human or vertebrae
(3 semester hours), General Chemistry w/Lab
(8 semester hours), Organic Chemistry w/Lab
(8 semester hours), Physics (8 semester hours),
Calculus (3 semester hours), Speech: public
speaking/communications (3 semester hours),
Economics: general, micro, or macro (3 semester
hours), General Education Electives: to be divided
among the social sciences, humanities, fine arts,
foreign language, business, or computer science
(12 semester hours), Statistic (3), General
Psychology (3).

College of Notre Dame of Maryland School of Pharmacy

4701 N. Charles Street, Baltimore, MD 21210
Phone: 410-435-0100;
Website: www.ndm.edu/admission/schoolofphar-
macy/
General Info: College of Notre Dame SOP is a pri-
vate school with an acceptance rate of 36.8% to
its pharmacy school **Male/Female Ratio:** 35/65
Class Size: 70 **Joint Degrees Offered:** None **PCAT**

required: Yes **PharmCAS required:** Yes **Minimum
GPA:** 2.5 **Average GPA:** 3.15 **Application
deadline:** February 1 **Application fee:** $55
In-State Tuition: $29,680 **Out-of-State Tuition:**
$29,680 **Pre-requisites:** General Chemistry
w/ lab (8 semesters), Organic Chemistry w/
lab (8 semesters), General Biology w/lab (8
semesters), Physiology or Anatomy & Physiology
(8 semesters); Microbiology (4 semesters),
Physics (3 semester hours), Calculus (3 semester
hours), Statistics (3 semester hours), Psychology
or Sociology (6 semester hours), Speech (3
semester hours), English Comp. (6 semester hours), Economics (3 semester hours),
Humanities (6 semester hours); Ethics (3 semester hours)

Concordia University Wisconsin School of Pharmacy

12800 N. Lake Shore Drive, Mequon, WI 53097
Phone: (262) 243-2755
Website: www.cuw.edu/pharmacy
General Info: Concordia University is a private
school **Male/Female Ratio:** 45/55 **Students
per Class:** 70-80 **Joint Degrees Offered:** N/A
PCAT: Required **PharmCAS:** Required **Minimum
GPA:** 2.7 **Average GPA:** 3.4 **Application
Deadline:** March 1 **Application Fee:** $50 **In-State
Tuition:** $27,840 **Out-of-State Tuition:** $27,840
Prerequisites: English Composition/Writing (3
semester hours), Biology I & II w/lab (8 semester
hours), Physics I & II w/ lab (8 semester hours),
General Chemistry I & II w/ lab (8 semester
hours), Organic Chemistry I & II w/ lab (8 semester hours), Calculus (4 semester hours), Statistics
(3 semester hours), General or Health Economics
(3 semester hours), Public Speaking (3 semester
hours), General electives (24 semester hours)

Creighton University Medical Center School of Pharmacy and Health Professionals

2500 California Plaza, Omaha, NE 68178
Phone: (402) 280-2662 **Fax:** (402) 280-5738
Website: www.spahp.creighton.edu/pharmacyde-
partment.asp
General Info: Private school with an accep-
tance rate of 14.3% to pharmacy school
Pharmacy Student Body: 683 **Male/Female
Ratio:** 35/65 **Students per Class:** 165 **Joint
Degrees Offered:** PharmD/MS, PharmD/MBA,

PharmD/PhD **PCAT:** Required **Minimum Score:** 60%. **PharmCAS:** Required **Minimum GPA:** 3.25 **Average GPA:** 3.43 **Application Deadline:** February 1 **Application Fee:** $60 **In-State Tuition:** $28,874 **Out-of-State Tuition:** $28,874 **Prerequisites:** English (6 semester hours), Biology I and II w/Labs (8 semester hours), General Chemistry I and II w/Labs (8 semester hours), Organic Chemistry I and II w/Labs (8 semester hours), Calculus (3 semester hours), Speech/Public Speaking (3 semester hours), Economics: micro or macro (3 semester hours), Electives (21 semester hours): 9 semester hours from Humanities or Behavioral or Social Sciences. Creighton undergraduates must complete 6 semester hours of Theology among the elective hours, Human Anatomy (3), Psychology (3).

Drake University College of Pharmacy and Health Sciences

2507 University Avenue, Cine Hall Suite 106, Des Moines, IA 50311
Phone: (800) 44-DRAKE **Fax:** (515) 271-4171
Website: www.drake.edu/cphs
General Info: Private school with an acceptance rate of 20% to pharmacy school **Pharmacy Student Body:** 503 **Male/Female Ratio:** 39/61 **Students per Class:** 100 **Joint Degrees Offered:** PharmD/MBA, PharmD/MPA, PharmD/JD **PCAT:** Required **Minimum Score:** 50%. **PharmCAS:** Required **Minimum GPA:** 3.0. **Average GPA:** 3.7 **Application Deadline:** December 1 **Application Fee:** None specified. **In-State Tuition:** $24,900 **Out-of-State Tuition:** $24,900 **Prerequisites:** English Composition (6 semester hours), Inorganic Chemistry w/Lab (8 semester hours), Organic Chemistry w/Lab (8 semester hours), Biology w/Lab (8 semester hours), Microbiology (3 semester hours), Calculus (3 semester hours), Statistics (3 semester hours), Public Speaking (3 semester hours).

Duquesne University of Mylan School of Pharmacy

306 Bayer Learning Center, Pittsburgh, PA 15282-1504
Phone: (412) 396-6377 **Fax:** (412) 296-1810
Website: www.pharmacy.duq.edu
General Info: Private school with an acceptance rate of 22.2% to pharmacy school. **Pharmacy**

Student Body: 959 **Male/Female Ratio:** 35/65 **Students per Class:** 227 **Joint Degrees Offered:** PharmD/MBA, PharmD/PhD, PharmD/MS **PCAT:** Not required **PharmCAS:** Not Required **Minimum GPA:** N/A **Average GPA:** 3.8 **Application Deadline:** December 1 **Application Fee:** $50 **In-State Tuition:** $22,454 **Out-of-State Tuition:** $22,454 **Prerequisites:** General Biology I and II w/Lab, General Chemistry I and II, Organic Chemistry I and II, Calculus I, General Physics I and II, English Composition and Literature, English Literature, Religious Studies, Philosophy, Modern U.S., European, or World History, Music or Art Appreciation, Economics, Statistics, Speech or Interpersonal Communication, Psychology, General Sociology. A minimum cumulative GPA average of 2.5 and no grade lower than "C" in each of the required courses is a minimum academic requirement to enter the professional phase of the pharmacy degree program.

D'Youville School of Pharmacy

320 Porter Avenue, Buffalo, NY 14201
Phone: (716) 829-8440
Website: www.dyc.edu/academics/pharmacy
General Info: D'Youville College is a private school **Male/Female Ratio:** 54/46 **Students per Class:** 65 **Joint Degrees Offered:** N/A **PCAT:** Required **PharmCAS:** Required **Minimum GPA:** 2.5 **Average GPA:** 3.2 **Application Deadline:** March 1 **Application Fee:** $50 **In-State Tuition:** Not given **Out-of-State Tuition:** Not given **Prerequisites:** English Composition I & II (6 semester hours), Biology I & II w/ lab (8 semester hours), Microbiology w/lab or Anatomy and Physiology w/ lab (4 semester hours), Physics I & II w/ lab (8 semester hours), General Chemistry I & II w/ lab (8 semester hours), Organic Chemistry I & II w/ lab (8 semester hours), Calculus (4 semester hours), Statistics (4 semester hours), General or Health Economics (3 semester hours), Public Speaking (3 semester hours), U.S. History (3 semester hours), Social Sciences (3 semester hours), Humanities (3 semester hours)

East Tennessee State University Bill Gatton College of Pharmacy

P.O. Box 70720, Johnson City, TN 37614
Phone: (423) 439-6300
Email: pharmacy@etsu.edu
Website: www.dev.etsu.edu/pharmacy/
General Info: Public school. Students per class: 80. **Joint Degrees Offered:** None **PCAT:** Required. **Minimum Score:** 65% **Average GPA:** 3.49 **Application Deadline:** TBA **Application Fee:** TBA. **In-State Tuition:** $19,500 **Out-of-State Tuition:** $22,884. **Prerequisites:** Chemistry w/Lab (8 semester hours), Organic Chemistry w/Lab (8 semester hours), Physics w/Lab (4 semester hours), Biology w/Lab (8 semester hours), Calculus (3 semester hours), Probability Statistics (3 semester hours), Communication Skills (9 semester hours; minimum of 3 semester hours Composition/Writing), Elective Courses (20 semester hours). Minimum total of 63 semester hours, Economics (3 semester hours), Microbiology (3), Other Biology (3).

Ferris State University College of Pharmacy

220 Ferris Drive, Big Rapids, MI 49307
Phone: (231) 591-2254 **Fax:** (231) 591-3829
General Info: Private school with an acceptance rate of 20% to pharmacy school. **Pharmacy Student Body:** 486. **Male/Female Ratio:** 48/52. **Students per Class:** 150. **Joint Degrees Offered:** PharmD/MBA **PCAT:** Required. **Minimum Score:** 80% **PharmCAS:** Not required **Minimum GPA:** 3.4 **Average GPA:** 3.7 **Application Deadline:** January 31 **Application Fee:** None specified. **Prerequisites:** General Chemistry (8–10 semester hours), Organic Chemistry (8–10 semester hours), General Biology (8 semester hours), Calculus for Life Sciences or Calculus (3–4 semester hours), English Composition (6 semester hours), Interpersonal Communication of Principles of Public Speaking (3 semester hours), Introduction to Psychology or Sociology (3 semester hours), Principles of Economics: Macroeconomics (3 semester hours), Cultural Enrichment (i.e. Humanities): one course must be at the 200+ level (9 semester hours).

Florida Agricultural and Mechanical University College of Pharmacy and Pharmaceutical Sciences

New Pharmacy Building, Room 333, 1415 S. Martin Luther King Jr. Boulevard, Tallahassee, FL 32307
Phone: (850) 599-3301 **Fax:** (850) 599-3347
Website: www.famu.edu
General Info: Public school with an acceptance rate of 21.7% to pharmacy school **Pharmacy Student Body:** 1,173 **Male/Female Ratio:** 30/70. **Students per Class:** 126 **Joint Degrees Offered:** None. **PCAT:** Not required **PharmCAS:** Not required. **Average GPA:** 3.3. **Application Deadline:** February 1 **Application Fee:** $20 **In-State Tuition:** $2,852 **Out-of-State Tuition:** $14,949 **Prerequisites:** None

Hampton University School of Pharmacy

Hampton, VA 23668
Phone: (757) 727-5071 **Fax:** (757) 727-5840
Website: www.hampton.edu
General Info: Private school with an acceptance rate of 24.4% to pharmacy school. **Pharmacy Student Body:** 361 **Male/Female Ratio:** 28/72 **Students per Class:** 68. **Joint Degrees Offered:** None **PharmCAS:** Not Required **Maximum GPA:** 2.75 **Average GPA:** 3.2 **Application Deadline:** March 1 **Application Fee:** $25 **In-State Tuition:** $15,318 **Out-of-State Tuition:** $12,600 **Prerequisites:** General Chemistry I and II (8 semester hours), English (6 semester hours), General Biology (8 semester hours), Calculus (3 semester hours), Speech (3 semester hours), Social Science Elective (3 semester hours), Organic Chemistry (8 semester hours), Physics w/Lab (10 semester hours), Humanities (6 semester hours), History I and II (6 semester hours), Physical Education (2 semester hours).

Harding University College of Pharmacy

915 E. Market Avenue, Box 12230; Searcy, AR 72149
Phone: 501-279-5205;
Website: www.harding.edu/Pharmacy
General Info: HU is a private school with an acceptance rate of 44.4% to its pharmacy school **Male/Female Ratio:** 45/55 **Class Size:** 60 **Joint Degrees Offered:** None **PCAT required:**

Yes **PharmCAS required:** Yes **Minimum GPA:** 2.7 **Average GPA:** 3.35 **Early admissions:** No **Application deadline:** February 1 **Application fee:** $50 **In-State Tuition:** $27,300 **Out-of-State Tuition:** $27,300 **Pre-requisites:** General Chemistry w/lab (8 semesters), Organic Chemistry w/lab (8 semesters), Cell Biology (4 semesters), Biochemistry (3 semesters), Physiology or Anatomy & Physiology (8 semesters); Microbiology (4 semesters), Zoology or Biology (3 semester hours), Physics (4 semester hours), Calculus (4 semester hours), Statistics (3 semester hours), Psychology or Sociology (3 semester hours), Speech (3 semester hours), English Comp. (3 semester hours), Economics (3 semester hours), Humanities (6 semester hours)

Howard University College of Pharmacy, Nursing, and Allied Health

2300 4th Street NW, Washington, DC 20054
Phone: (202) 806-4636 **Fax:** (202) 234-1375
Website: www.howard.edu
General Info: Private school with an acceptance rate of 9.8% to pharmacy school. **Pharmacy Student Body:** 371 **Male/Female Ratio:** 47/50 **Students per Class:** 121 **Joint Degrees Offered:** PharmD/MBA **PCAT:** Required **Minimum Score:** 40% **PharmCAS:** Required **Minimum GPA:** 2.5 **Average GPA:** 3.2 **Early Admissions Deadline:** September 1 **Application Deadline:** December 1 **Application Fee:** $45 **In-State Tuition:** $13,040 **Out-of-State Tuition:** $13,040 **Prerequisites:** English (6 semester hours), General Chemistry w/Lab (10 semester hours), General Biology: microbiology or anatomy/physiology can be used in place of Biology II course (6 semester hours), Organic Chemistry w/Lab (9 semester hours), Calculus (4 semester hours), Physics w/Lab (10 semester hours), Speech (3 semester hours), Humanities: may include art, music, literature, drama, theatre, religion, philosophy, medical terminology, foreign language (6 semester hours), Socio-behavioral Sciences: may include sociology, psychology, anthropology, economics, history, philosophy, political science, medical, and government (6 semester hours), General Electives: may include statistics, computer fundamentals, mathematics above Calculus I, additional humanities, and/or socio-behavioral sciences (9 semester hours).

Husson University School of Pharmacy

One College Circle, Bangor, ME 04401
Phone: (207) 973-2029
Website: www.husson.edu
General Info: Husson University is a private school **Male/Female Ratio:** 54/46 **Students per Class:** 65 **Joint Degrees Offered:** N/A **PCAT:** Required **PharmCAS:** Required **Minimum GPA:** 2.7 **Average GPA:** 3.5 **Application Deadline:** March 1 **Application Fee:** $50 **In-State Tuition:** $13,140 **Out-of-State Tuition:** $13,140 **Prerequisites:** English Composition (6 semester hours), Biology I & II w/lab (8 semester hours), Anatomy & Physiology w/lab (8 semester hours), General Chemistry I & II w/lab (8 semester hours), Organic Chemistry I & II w/ lab (8 semester hours), Calculus (4 semester hours), Statistics (3 semester hours), General or Health Economics (3 semester hours), Public Speaking (3 semester hours), Psychology or Sociology (3 semester hours), General electives (6 semester hours)

Idaho State University College of Pharmacy

P.O. Box 8288, 970 S. 5th Street, Pocatello, ID 83209
Phone: (208) 282-2175 **Fax:** (208) 282-4482
Website: http://pharmacy.isu.edu/live
General Info: State school with an acceptance rate of 12.5% to pharmacy school **Pharmacy Student Body:** 226 **Male/Female Ratio:** 52/48 **Students per Class:** 61 **Joint Degrees Offered:** PharmD/MBA, PharmD/MS, PharmD/PhD **PCAT:** Not required **PharmCAS:** Not required **Minimum GPA:** 2.50 **Average GPA:** 3.61 **Application Deadline:** February 1 **Application Fee:** $55 **In-State Tuition:** $12.620 **Out-of-State Tuition:** $25,744 **Prerequisites:** General Biology (4 semester credits), General Chemistry I and II w/Lab (9 semester credits), Calculus (4 semester credits), Organic Chemistry I and II w/Lab (8 semester credits), General Physics I (no Lab required) credits, General Microbiology w/Lab (4 semester credits), Economics (3 semester credits), Anatomy and Physiology I and II w/Lab (8 semester hours) or Human Anatomy w/Lab and Human Physiology w/Lab, Human Anatomy w/Lab and Cell Biology w/Lab, Human Anatomy w/Lab, Genetics, English Composition, Public Speaking, Humanities.

Lake Erie College of Osteopathic Medicine School of Pharmacy

1858 W. Grandview Boulevard, Erie, PA 16509
Phone: (814) 866-6641 **Fax:** (814) 866-8123
Website: http://lecom.edu
General Info: Private School with an acceptance rate of 9% to pharmacy school **Pharmacy Student Body:** 367 **Male/Female Ratio:** 33/66 **Students per Class:** 130 **Student/Faculty Ratio:** 9/1. **Joint Degrees Offered:** None **PharmCAS:** Required **Minimum GPA:** 2.70 **Average GPA:** 3.56 **Application Deadline:** March 1 **Application Fee:** $50 **In-State Tuition:** $21,000 **Out-of-State Tuition:** $22,200 **Prerequisites:** English (6 semester hours), Biology w/Lab (8 semester hours), Inorganic Chemistry w/Lab (8 semester hours), Organic Chemistry w/Lab (8 semester hours), Physics (8 semester hours), Psychology or Sociology (6 semester hours).
*Satellite campus—Bradenton (4-year program); Erie (3-year accelerated)

Lipscomb University College of Pharmacy

One University Park Drive, Nashville, TN 37204
Phone: 615-966-7160
Website: http://pharmacy.lipscomb.edu
General Information: Lipscomb University is a private school with an acceptance rate of 37.5% to its program; **Male/Female Ratio:** 27/73 **Class Size:** 75; Joint **Degrees Offered:** None **PCAT required:** Yes **PharmCAS required:** Yes **Minimum GPA:** 2.5 **Average GPA:** 3.38 **Early admissions:** No **Application deadline:** February 1 **Application fee:** $50 **In-State Tuition:** $28,875 **Out-of-State Tuition:** $28,875 **Pre-requisites:** General Chemistry w/ lab (8 semesters), Organic Chemistry w/lab (8 semesters), Physics (4 semester hours), Calculus (3 semester hours), Statistics (3 semester hours), Speech (3 semester hours), English Comp. (6 semester hours), Economics (3 semester hours), Humanities (6 semester hours)

Loma Linda University School of Pharmacy

West Hall #1316, 11262 Campus Street, Loma Linda, CA 92350
Phone: (909) 558-1300 **Fax:** (909) 558-4859
Website: www.llu.edu

General Info: Private school with an acceptance rate of 6.1% to pharmacy school. **Pharmacy Student Body:** 189 **Male/Female Ratio:** 33/67 **Students per Class:** 61 **Joint Degrees Offered:** None **PCAT:** Required **PharmCAS:** Not required **Average GPA:** 3.3 **Minimum GPA:** 2.75 **Application Deadline:** December 15 **Application Fee:** $60. **In-State Tuition:** $30,600 **Out-of-State Tuition:** $30,600 **Prerequisites:** Sciences: General Chemistry w/Lab (1 year), Organic Chemistry w/Lab (1 year), General Biology of Zoology w/Lab (1 year), General Physics w/Lab (1 year), Anatomy (1 semester or 1 quarter), Mathematics: Calculus (1 semester or 2 quarters), Computer Proficiency, General Education: English Composition and Speech (9 semester hours), Humanities/Fine Arts (12 semester hours), Behavioral Sciences (12 semester hours). A one-year course with laboratory is considered to be 8 semester hours.

Long Island University Arnold and Marie Schwartz College of Pharmacy and Health Services

75 DeKalb Avenue, At University Plaza, Brooklyn, NY 11201
Phone: (718) 488-1004 **Fax:** (718) 488-0628
Website: www.liu.edu
General Info: Private school with an acceptance rate of 9.1% to pharmacy school. **Pharmacy Student Body:** 226 **Male/Female Ratio:** 39/61 **Joint Degrees Offered:** None **PCAT:** N/A. **PharmCAS:** Required **Minimum GPA:** 3.0 **Average GPA:** Not specified **Early Admissions Deadline:** September 1 **Application Deadline:** February 12 **Application Fee:** $30. Upon acceptance to the P-3, Pharm.D. program, applicants expected to pay $500 to secure their spot.
In-State Tuition: $27,452 **Out-of-State Tuition:** $27,452 **Prerequisites:** General Chemistry I and II (8 semester hours), General Biology I and II (8 semester hours), Organic Chemistry I and II (8 semester hours), Physics (4 semester hours), Human Anatomy (4 semester hours), Precalculus (4 semester hours), English Composition (3 semester hours), English Literature (12 semester hours), General Psychology (3 semester hours), History or Philosophy (6 semester hours), Economics: micro or macro (3 semester hours), Calculus, Philosophy, Psychology, Speech.

Massachusetts College of Pharmacy and Health Sciences—Boston

179 Longwood Avenue, Boston, MA 02115
Phone: (617) 732-2800 **Fax:** (617) 732-2801
Website: www.mcphs.edu
General Info: Private school with an acceptance rate of 67% for freshman, 20% for transfers to pharmacy school. **Pharmacy Student Body:** 1,554. **Male/Female Ratio:** 29/71. **Students per Class:** 296. **Joint Degrees Offered:** None **PCAT:** Required. **Minimum Score:** 80% **PharmCAS:** required. **Minimum GPA:** None specified **Average GPA:** 3.53. **Application Deadline:** February 1 **Application Fee:** $70 **In-State Tuition:** $25,000 **Out-of-State Tuition:** $25,000 **Prerequisites:** Required: Biology General and Human w/Labs (12 semester hours), Microbiology w/Lab (4 semester hours), General Chemistry w/Lab (12 semester hours), Organic Chemistry w/Lab (12 semester hours), English Composition (9 semester hours), Sociology (4 semester hours), Probability Statistics (4 semester hours), Physics w/Lab (6 semester hours), Economics: macro, micro, or general (4 semester hours), Electives: Humanities (4 semester hours), Social Sciences (4 semester hours), Behavioral Sciences (4 semester hours), Mathematics or Computer Science (4 semester hours), Calculus.

Massachusetts College of Pharmacy and Health Sciences—Worcester, MA and Manchester, NH

19 Foster Street, Suite 400, Worchester, MA 01608
Phone: (580) 890-8855 ext. 1911 **Fax:** (508) 890-8515 **Website:** www.mcphs.edu
General Info: Private school with an acceptance rate of 20% to pharmacy school. **Pharmacy Student Body:** 480 **Male/Female Ratio:** 34/66. **Students per Class:** 190 **Joint Degrees Offered:** None. **PCAT:** Required. **Minimum Score:** 80%. **PharmCAS:** Not required. **Minimum GPA:** None specified. **Average GPA:** 3.38 **Early Admissions Deadline:** September 1 **Application Deadline:** Feb. 1 **Application Fee:** $70. **In-State Tuition:** $38,100 **Out-of-State Tuition:** $38,100 **Prerequisites:** Required: Biology General and Human w/Labs (12 quarter hours), Microbiology w/Lab (4 quarter hours), General Chemistry w/Lab (12 quarter hours), Organic Chemistry w/Lab (12 quarter hours), English Composition (9 quarter hours), Introduction to Psychology (4 quarter hours), Introduction to Sociology (4 quarter hours), Introduction to History and Political Science (4 quarter hours), Calculus (4 quarter hours), Probability Statistics (4 quarter hours), Physics w/Lab (6 quarter hours), Economics: macro, micro, or general (4 quarter hours), Electives: Humanities (4 quarter hours), Social Sciences, Behavioral Sciences (4 quarter hours), Mathematics or Computer Science (4 quarter hours)
*The Worcester, MA and Manchester, NH campuses offer accelerated programs designed exclusively for transfer students. The Manchester, NH campus is a satellite of the Worcester, MA campus and shares full-accredited status through the Worcester program.

Mercer University College of Pharmacy and Health Sciences

3001 Mercer University Drive, Atlanta, GA 30341-4155
Phone: (678) 547-6304 **Fax:** (678) 547-6315
Website: www.cophs.mercer.edu
General Info: Private school with an acceptance rate of 7.7% to pharmacy school. **Pharmacy Student Body:** 556 **Male/Female Ratio:** 35/65 **Students per Class:** 147 **Joint Degrees Offered:** PharmD/MBA, PharmD/PhD **PCAT:** Required **Minimum Score:** 60%. **PharmCAS:** Required **Minimum GPA:** 2.80. **Average GPA:** 3.51 **Application Deadline:** January 5 **Application Fee:** $25 **In-State Tuition:** $24,523 **Out-of-State Tuition:** $24,523 **Prerequisites:** General Chemistry (8 semester hours), Organic Chemistry (8 semester hours), General Biology or Zoology (8 semester hours), Physics (4 semester hours), Calculus (3–4 semester hours), English Composition (6 semester hours), Speech (3 semester hours), Humanities Electives (6 semester hours), Economics (3 semester hours), Social/Behavioral Sciences (6 semester hours), Other Electives (to total 6 semester hours).

Midwestern University Chicago College of Pharmacy

55 31st Street, Downers Grove, IL 60515
Phone: 630-515-6171 **Fax:** 630-971-6097
Website: http://www.midwestern.edu/ccp
General Info: Private school and it has an accep-

tance rate of 17.5% to its pharmacy school. **Pharmacy School Student Body:** 811. **Male/Female Ratio:** 39/61 **Students per Class:** 202 **Joint Degrees Offered:** None **PCAT:** Required **PharmCAS:** Required **Minimum GPA:** 2.50 **Average GPA:** 3.33 **Early Admissions:** Not offered **Application Deadline:** January 5 (PharmCAS), March 1 (Supplemental) **Application fee:** $50 **In-State Tuition:** $23,006 **Out-of-State Tuition:** $25,050 **Prerequisites:** English Composition (6 semester hours), Biology w/lab (8 semester hours), Human or Vertebrate Anatomy (3 semester hours), General Chemistry w/lab (8 semester hours), Organic Chemistry w/lab (8 semester hours), Physics (6 semester hours), Calculus (3 semester hours), Speech/public speaking (3 semester hours), Economics (3 semester hours), General Education Electives (11 semester hours), Statistics, Social and Behavioral Studies.

Midwestern University College of Pharmacy, Glendale

19555 N. 59th Avenue, Glendale, AZ 85308 **Phone:** (623) 572-3500 **Fax:** (623) 752-3510 **Website:** www.midwestern.edu/Pages/CPG.html **General Info:** Private school with an acceptance rate of 13.9% to pharmacy school. **Pharmacy Student Body:** 389 **Male/Female Ratio:** 55/45 **Students per Class:** 129 **Joint Degrees Offered:** None. **PCAT:** Required **PharmCAS:** Required **Minimum GPA:** 2.5 **Average GPA:** 3.45 **Application Deadline:** January 5 **Application Fee:** $50. **In-State Tuition:** $23,258 **Out-of-State Tuition:** $23,258 **Prerequisites:** English Composition (6 semester hours), Biology w/Lab (8 semester hours), Human or Vertebrate Anatomy (3 semester hours), General Chemistry w/Lab (8 semester hours), Organic Chemistry w/Lab (8 semester hours), Physics (6 semester hours), Calculus (3 semester hours), Speech/Public Speaking (3 semester hours), Economics (3 semester hours), General Education Electives (11 semester hours), Social Sciences (6 hours).

Nesbitt College of Pharmacy and Nursing at Wilkes University

Wilkes-Barre, PA 18766 **Phone:** (570) 408-4280 **Fax:** (570) 408-7828 **Website:** www.wilkes.edu/pharm **General Info:** Private school with an acceptance

rate of 23.8% to pharmacy school. **Pharmacy Student Body:** 269 **Male/Female Ratio:** 36/64 **Students per Class:** 64 **Joint Degrees Offered:** PharmD/MBA, PharmD/PhD, PharmD/MS **PCAT:** Required **PharmCAS:** Not required **Minimum GPA:** 2.0 **Average GPA:** 3.2 **Application Deadline:** February 1 **Application Fee:** N/A **In-State Tuition:** $23,200 **Out-of-State Tuition:** $23,200 **Prerequisites:** To learn more about the prerequisites for the school, visit their website at www.wilkes.edu/pages/463.asp to contact the school directly.

North Dakota State University College of Pharmacy

123 Sudro Hall, Fargo, ND 58105-5055 **Phone:** (701) 231-7609 **Fax:** (701) 231-7606 **Website:** www.ndsu.edu/pharmacy **General Info:** State school with an acceptance rate of 49.8% to pharmacy school. **Pharmacy Student Body:** 344 **Male/Female Ratio:** 48/52 **Students per Class:** 85 **Joint Degrees Offered:** Pharm.D./M.B.A., Pharm.D./Ph.D. **PCAT:** Required **PharmCAS:** Not required **Minimum GPA:** 3.00 **Average GPA:** 3.86 **Application Deadline:** January 1 **Application Fee:** $100 **In-State Tuition:** $4,774 **Out-of-State Tuition:** $12,747 **Prerequisites:** General Chemistry I and II (6 semester credits), Organic Chemistry I and II (6 semester credits), Cellular Biology (3 semester credits), Biology: Anatomy and Physiology I and II (6–8 semester credits), Physics (3 semester credits), Calculus I and II (8 semester credits), English Composition I and II (6 semester credits), Economics (3 semester credits), Microbiology (2–3 semester credits), Humanities and Fine Arts (6 semester credits), Social Sciences (3 semester credits), Wellness (2 semester credits).

Northeastern Ohio Universities College of Pharmacy (NEOUCOM)

4209 Street, Route 44, P.O. Box 95, Rootstown, OH 44272-0095 **Phone:** (330) 325-6270 **Website:** www.neoucom.edu/audience/applicants/succeed/admi/Pharmadmission **General Info:** Public school. The school's program is a new program. **Pharmacy Student Body:** 300 expected **Joint Degrees Offered:** None **PCAT:** Required **Minimum Score:** 50% **PharmCAS:**

Required **Minimum GPA:** 2.5 **Average GPA:**
5.25 **Early Admissions Deadline:** September 1
Application Deadline: February 1 **Application
Fee:** $50 **In-State Tuition:** $16,760 **Out-of-State
Tuition:** $29,500 **Prerequisites:** Principles of
Biology w/Lab (8 semester hours), Principles of
Chemistry w/Lab (8 semester hours), Organic
Chemistry w/Lab (8 semester hours), General
Physics (6 semester hours), Biochemistry
(6 semester hours), Calculus (3 semester
hours), Statistics (3 semester hours), English
Composition/Literature (6 semester hours),
Economics (3 semester hours), Computer Literacy
(3 semester hours), Speech/Communication
(3 semester hours), Psychology (3 semester
hours), Social Science Electives (6 semester
hours), Humanities Electives (6 semester hours).
Total of 72 semester hours needed.

Northeastern University Bouvé College of Health and Sciences School of Pharmacy

360 Huntington Avenue, 206 Mugar, Boston, MA
02115
Phone: (617) 373-2000 **Fax:** (617) 373-7655
Website: www.bouve.neu.edu/pharmacy
General Info: Private school with an acceptance rate
of 10.6% to pharmacy school. **Pharmacy Student
Body:** 695. **Male/Female Ratio:** 36/64. **Students
per Class:** 142. **Joint Degrees Offered:** None.
PCAT: Required. **Minimum Score:** 80%. **PharmCAS:**
Not required. **Minimum GPA:** None specified.
Average GPA: 3.8. **Application Deadline:** January
15 **Application Fee:** $50 **In-State Tuition:** $29,910
Out-of-State Tuition: $29,910 **Prerequisites:**
Biology w/Labs (2 semesters), Chemistry w/Labs
(2 semesters), Calculus (1 semester), Organic
Chemistry w/Lab (2 semesters), Microbiology
w/Lab (1 semester), Biochemistry (1 semester),
Psychology (1 semester), English (1 semester),
Anatomy and Physiology w/Lab (2 semesters),
Economics (1 semester), Social Sciences
(2 semesters), Humanities (2 semesters).

Nova Southeastern University College of Pharmacy

3200 S. University Drive, Ft. Lauderdale, FL
33328
Phone: (954) 262-1101; **Fax:** (954) 262-3995;
Website: http://pharmacy.nova.edu/home.html
General Info: Private school with an acceptance

rate of 16.7% to pharmacy school. **Pharmacy
Student Body:** 807. **Male/Female Ratio:** 40/60.
Students per Class: 197. **Joint Degrees Offered:**
PharmD/MBA **PCAT:** Required. **PharmCAS:**
Required. **Minimum GPA:** 2.75. **Average
GPA:** 3.40. **Application Deadline:** January 5.
Application Fee: $50. **In-State Tuition:** $22,545.
Out-of-State Tuition: $26,666. **Prerequisites:**
English (6 semester hours), General Chemistry w/
Lab (8 semester hours), Organic Chemistry
w/Lab (8 semester hours), General Biology
(3 semester hours), Anatomy and Physiology
(3 semester hours), General Biology or Anatomy
and Physiology: in addition to previous prerequisites, must include a one-hour lab (4 semester
hours), Calculus (3 semester hours), Statistics
(3 semester hours), Speech (3 semester
hours), Macroeconomics (3 semester hours),
Microeconomics (3 semester hours), Social/
Behavioral Sciences/Humanities: must have
3 hours in social/behavioral sciences and
3 hours in humanities; remaining 9 hours can be
in either discipline (15 semester hours).

Ohio Northern University College of Pharmacy

Roberts-Evans, 525 S. Main Street, Ada, OH
45810
Phone: (419) 772-2277 **Fax:** (419) 772-2720
Website: www.onu.edu/pharmacy
General Info: Private school with an acceptance
rate of 21.7% to pharmacy school. **Pharmacy
Student Body:** 1,002 **Male/Female Ratio:**
36/64. **Students per Class:** 169 **Joint Degrees
Offered:** PharmD/JD, Pharmacy/Biology Dial
PCAT: Not required. **PharmCAS:** Not required.
Minimum GPA: N/A **Average GPA:** 3.78
Application Deadline: November 1. **Application
Fee:** $30. **In-State Tuition:** $31,545 **Out-of-
State Tuition:** $31,545 **Prerequisites:** General
Chemistry, Organic Chemistry, Biology, Zoology,
Calculus.

Ohio State University College of Pharmacy

500 W. 12th Avenue, Columbus, OH 43210
Phone: (614) 292-5711 **Fax:** (614) 292-3113
Website: www.pharmacy.ohio-state.edu
General Info: Public school with an acceptance
rate of 16.7% to pharmacy school. **Pharmacy
Student Body:** 459. **Male/Female Ratio:** 40/60

Students per Class: 120. **Joint Degrees Offered:** PharmD/MS, PharmD/MBA, PharmD/PhD **PCAT:** Required **Minimum Score:** 50% **PharmCAS:** Required **Minimum GPA:** 3.0 **Average GPA:** 3.6 **Application Deadline:** December 1 **Application Fee:** U.S. applicants: $40; international applicants: $50 **In-State Tuition:** $12,693 **Out-of-State Tuition:** $14,205 **Prerequisites:** Human Anatomy w/Lab (3 semester hours), General Chemistry w/Lab (10 semester hours), Analytical Chemistry w/Lab (3 semester hours), Organic Chemistry w/Lab (8 semester hours), General Biology w/Lab (3 semester hours), Calculus I and II (10 semester hours), Microbiology w/Lab (3 semester hours), General Physics w/Lab (10 semester hours), General Education/Liberal Education (30 semester hours).

Oregon State University College of Pharmacy

203 Pharmacy Building, Corvallis, OR 97331-3507 **Phone:** (541) 737-3424 **Fax:** (541) 737-3999 **Website:** http://pharmacy.oregonstate.edu **General Info:** Public school with an acceptance rate of 8.6% to pharmacy school **Pharmacy Student Body:** 328 **Male/Female Ratio:** 49/51 **Students per Class:** 87 **Joint Degrees Offered:** PharmD/MBA, PharmD/PhD **PCAT:** Not required. **PharmCAS:** Required. **Minimum GPA:** In-state: 2.75 out-of-state: 3.0 **Average GPA:** 3.54 **Early Admissions Deadline:** September 1 **Application Deadline:** December 1 **Application Fee:** $100 **In-State Tuition:** $18,935 **Out-of-State Tuition:** $23,049 **Prerequisites:** English I and II (6 quarter hours), General Chemistry w/Lab (15 quarter hours), Organic Chemistry w/Lab (12 quarter hours), Principles of Biology w/Lab (12 quarter hours), Cell and Molecular Biology (4 quarter hours), Microbiology w/Lab (5 quarter hours), Calculus (4 quarter hours), Introduction to Statistics (3 quarter hours), Human Physiology of Biochemistry (12 quarter hours), General Physics w/Lab (15 quarter hours), General Psychology (3 quarter hours), Micro- or Macroeconomics (4 quarter hours), Interpersonal Communication (3 quarter hours), Human Anatomy.

Pacific University School of Pharmacy

2043 College Way, Forest Grove, OR 97116 **Phone:** (503) 352-3123 **Fax:** (503) 352-3158 **Website:** www.pacificu.edu/pharmd **General Info:** Private school. The school of pharmacy is a new program to the university; matriculation of the inaugural class is fall of 2006. **Joint Degrees Offered:** None **PCAT:** Not required **PharmCAS:** Not required **Minimum GPA:** 2.7 **Average GPA:** 3.4 **Class Size:** 96 **Male/Female Ratio:** 28/68 **Application Deadline:** December 1 **Application Fee:** $95 **In-State Tuition:** $24,523 **Out-of-State Tuition:** $36,556 **Prerequisites:** General Biology w/Lab (8 semester/12 quarter hours), Microbiology: lab not required (3 semester/3 quarter hours), Human Anatomy and Physiology w/Lab (8 semester/12 quarter hours), General Chemistry w/Lab (8 semester/12 quarter hours), Organic Chemistry w/Lab (8 semester/12 quarter hours), Physics w/Lab (3 semester/4 quarter hours), English Composition (6 semester/8 quarter hours), Psychology: intro or abnormal (3 semester/3 quarter hours), Economics: micro or macro (3 semester/3 quarter hours), Social/Behavioral Sciences (3 semester/3 quarter hours), Humanities/Fine Arts (3 semester/3 quarter hours), Mathematics (3 semester/quarter halves).

Palm Beach Atlantic University Lloyd L. Gregory School of Pharmacy

900 S. Olive Avenue, Palm Beach, FL 33401 **Phone:** (561) 803-2000 **Fax:** (561) 803-2703 **Website:** www.pba.edu **General Info:** Private school with an acceptance rate of 4.8% to pharmacy school **Pharmacy Student Body:** 257 **Male/Female Ratio:** 33/67. **Students per Class:** 78 **Joint Degrees Offered:** Pharm.D./M.B.A. **PCAT:** Required **PharmCAS:** Required. **Minimum GPA:** 2.75–3.00 **Average GPA:** 3.46 **Early Admissions Deadline:** September 1 **Application Deadline:** February 1 **Application Fee:** $75 **In-State Tuition:** $29,500 **Out-of-State Tuition:** $29,500 **Prerequisites:** English (6 semester hours), General Chemistry w/Lab (8 semester hours), Organic Chemistry w/Lab (8 semester hours), General Biology w/Lab (8 semester hours), Microbiology w/Lab (4 semester hours), Economics (3 semester hours), Calculus (4 semester hours), Elementary

Statistics (3 semester hours), Speech (3 semester hours), Humanities and/or Social/Behavioral Sciences (12 semester hours).

Philadelphia College of Osteopathic Medicine School of Pharmacy–Georgia Campus

625 Old Peachtree Rd., NW, Suwanee, GA 30024
Phone: (678) 407-7340
Website: www.pcom.edu
General Info: PCOM is a private school **Male/Female Ratio:** 44/56 **Students per Class:** 75
Joint Degrees Offered: N/A **PCAT:** Required
PharmCAS: Required **Minimum GPA:** 2.5
Average GPA: 3.1 **Application Deadline:** March 1
Application Fee: $50 **In-State Tuition:** $29,000
Out-of-State Tuition: $29,000 **Prerequisites:**
English Composition (6 semester hours), Biology I & II w/ lab (8 semester hours), Physics w/lab (4 semester hours), General Chemistry I & II w/lab (8 semester hours), Organic Chemistry I & II w/lab (8 semester hours), Calculus (4 semester hours), Statistics (3 semester hours), General or Health Economics (3 semester hours), Public Speaking (3 semester hours), Social/Behavioral Sciences (3 semester hours), Humanities (3 semester hours), Other electives (6 semester hours)

Presbyterian College School of Pharmacy

503 South Broad Street, Clinton, SC 29325
Phone: (864) 938-3911
Website: www.pharmacy.presby.edu
General Info: Presbyterian College is a private school **Male/Female Ratio:** 74/26 **Students per Class:** 80 **Joint Degrees Offered:** N/A **PCAT:** Required **PharmCAS:** Required **Minimum GPA:** 2.75 **Average GPA:** 3.25 **Application Deadline:** January 5 **Application Fee:** $60 **In-State Tuition:** $30,000 **Out-of-State Tuition:** $30,000 **Prerequisites:** English Composition (6 semester hours), Biology w/lab (8 semester hours), Microbiology w/lab (4 semester hours), Human Anatomy & Physiology (6 semester hours), Physics (3 semester hours), General Chemistry I & II w/lab (8 semester hours), Organic Chemistry I & II w/lab (8 semester hours), Calculus (3 semester hours), Statistics (3 semester hours), General or Health Economics (3 semester hours), Public Speaking (3 semester hours), Sociology or Psychology (3 semester hours), Ethics, Religion, or Philosophy

(3 semester hours), History or Political Science (3 semester hours)

Purdue University School of Pharmacy and Pharmaceutical Sciences

575 Stadium Mall Drive, West Lafayette, IN 47907
Phone: (765) 494-1368 **Fax:** (765) 494-7880
Website: www.pharmacy.purdue.edu
General Info: Public school with an acceptance rate of 15.2% to pharmacy school. **Pharmacy Student Body:** 640 **Male/Female Ratio:** 35/65
Student/Faculty Ratio: 9/1 **Joint Degrees Offered:** Pharm.D./Ph.D., Pharm.D./B.S., Pharm.D./M.S.I.A. **PCAT:** Not required **PharmCAS:** Required **Minimum GPA:** 3.2 out-of-state applicants. **Average GPA:** 3.60 **Application Deadline:** December 1 **Application Fee:** $5. **In-State Tuition:** $16,390 **Out-of-State Tuition:** $32,490
Prerequisites: General Biology (2 semesters), General Chemistry (2 semesters), Calculus (2 semesters), English (2 semesters), Anatomy/Physiology (2 semesters), Organic Chemistry (2 semesters), Physics (1 semester), Microbiology (1 semester), Economics (1 semester).

Regis University School of Pharmacy

3333 Regis Blvd., Denver, CO 80221
Phone: (303) 458-4344
Website: www.regis.edu/pharmD
General Info: Regis University is a private school **Male/Female Ratio:** 47/53 **Students per Class:** 75 **Joint Degrees Offered:** N/A **PCAT:** Required **PharmCAS:** Required **Minimum GPA:** 2.5 **Average GPA:** 3.2 **Application Deadline:** March 1 **Application Fee:** N/A **In-State Tuition:** $35,404 **Out-of-State Tuition:** $35,404 **Prerequisites:** English Composition (3 semester hours), Biology I & II w/lab (8 semester hours), Microbiology w/lab (4 semester hours), Human Anatomy & Physiology w/lab (8 semester hours), Physics (3 semester hours), General Chemistry I & II w/lab (8 semester hours), Organic Chemistry I & II w/lab (8 semester hours), Calculus (3 semester hours), General Economics (3 semester hours), Public Speaking (3 semester hours), Psychology (3 semester hours), Religious Studies (3 semester hours), Philosophy (3 semester hours), Sociology (3 semester hours), Social Science elective (3 semester hours), General Electives (5 semester hours)

Roosevelt University College of Pharmacy

1400 N. Roosevelt Blvd., Schaumburg, IL 60173
Phone: (847) 619-7287
Website: www.roosevelt.edu/pharmacy
General Info: Roosevelt University is a private
school **Male/Female Ratio:** N/A **Students per
Class:** 68 **Joint Degrees Offered:** N/A **PCAT:**
Required **PharmCAS:** Required **Minimum GPA:**
2.75 **Average GPA:** N/A **Application Deadline:**
December 1 **Application Fee:** $100 **In-State
Tuition:** $19,000 **Out-of-State Tuition:** $19,900
Prerequisites: English Composition I & II (6 semes-
ter hours), Biology I & II w/lab (8 semester hours),
Microbiology (3 semester hours), Human Anatomy
& Physiology w/lab (6 semester hours), Physics w/
lab (4 semester hours), General Chemistry I & II
w/lab (8 semester hours), Organic Chemistry I &
II w/lab (8 semester hours), Calculus (3 semester
hours), General Economics (3 semester hours),
Statistics (3 semester hours), Public Speaking
(3 semester hours), Humanities (6 semester
hours), Social and Behavioral Science (6 semester
hours)

Rosalind Franklin University of Medicine and Science, College of Pharmacy

3333 Green Bay Road, North Chicago, IL 60064
Phone: (847) 578-3204
Website: rosalindfranklin.edu/collegeofpharmacy
General Info: Rosalind Franklin University is a
private school **Male/Female Ratio:** N/A **Students
per Class:** N/A **Joint Degrees Offered:** N/A
PCAT: Required **PharmCAS:** Required **Minimum
GPA:** 2.75 **Average GPA:** N/A **Application
Deadline:** March 1 **Application Fee:** $50 **In-State
Tuition:** $28,000 **Out-of-State Tuition:** $28,900
Prerequisites: Written Communication (6 semes-
ter hours), Biology I & II w/lab (8 semester
hours), Anatomy or Physiology w/lab (4 semes-
ter hours), Physics w/lab (4 semester hours),
General Chemistry w/lab (8 semester hours),
Organic Chemistry w/lab (8 semester hours),
Calculus (3 semester hours), General Economics
(3 semester hours), Statistics (3 semester hours),
Public Speaking (3 semester hours), Humanities
(6 semester hours), Social Science (6 semester
hours), Behavioral Science (3 semester hours),
Electives (3 semester hours)

Rutgers, the State University of New Jersey Ernest Mario School of Pharmacy

William Levine Hall, 160 Frelinghuysen Road,
Piscataway, NJ 08854
Phone: (732) 445-2675 **Fax:** (732) 445-5767
Website: http://pharmacy.rutgers.edu
General Info: Public School with an acceptance
rate of 8.3% to pharmacy school. **Pharmacy
Student Body:** 1,331. **Male/Female Ratio:**
38/62. **Students per Class:** 291 **Joint Degrees
Offered:** None **PCAT:** Strongly recommended
PharmCAS: Not required **Minimum GPA:** 3.0
Average GPA: 3.43 **Application Deadline:**
January 15 **Application Fee:** $60 **In-State
Tuition:** $8,799 **Out-of-State Tuition:** $18,231
Prerequisites: General Biology I and II
(8 semester hours), General Chemistry I and II
(8 semester hours), Chemistry Lab (1 semester
hour), Calculus I (4 semester hours), English
Composition I and II or Public Speaking
(6 semester hours; at least 3 semester hours
must be English Composition), Organic Chemistry
I and II (8 semester hours), Organic Chemistry
Lab (2 semester hours), General Physics I and
II (8 semester hours), General Physics Lab
(1 semester hour), Systems Physiology
(3 semester hours; course content is exclusively
physiology; students who complete anatomy and
physiology courses must complete an Anatomy
and Physiology II course in order to satisfy the
requirement), Introduction to Microeconomics
(3 semester hours), Basic Statistics for Research
(3 semester hours).

St. John Fisher Wegmans School of Pharmacy

3690 East Avenue, Rochester, NY 14618
Phone: (585) 383-8172 **Email:** pharmacy@sjfc.
edu **Website:** www.sjfc.edu/pharmacy
General Info: Private school **Pharmacy Student
Body:** 55 students in its inaugural class of 2006.
Joint Degrees Offered: None **PCAT:** Required
Minimum GPA: 2.75 **Average GPA:** Not specified
Application Deadline: February 1 **Application
Fee:** $30 **In-State Tuition:** $28,500 **Out-of-State
Tuition:** $24,000 **Prerequisites:** Calculus
(4 semester hours), Statistics (3 semester hours),
General Chemistry w/Lab (8 semester hours),
Organic Chemistry w/Lab (8 semester hours),
Physics (4 semester hours), Biology w/Lab

(12 semester hours), English Composition/ Literature and Speech (9 semester hours; one must be English Composition and one course must be speech), Economics (3 semester hours; recommend micro- and/or macroeconomics), Humanities and/or Social/Behavioral Sciences (12 semester hours).

St. John's University College of Pharmacy and Allied Health Professionals

8000 Utopia Parkway, Jamaica, NY 11439
Phone: (718) 990-6411 **Fax:** (718) 990-1871
Website: http://new.stjohns.edu/academics/ graduate/pharmacy
General Info: Private school with an acceptance rate of 14.3% to pharmacy school. **Pharmacy Student Body:** 1,547 **Male/Female Ratio:** 37/63 **Students per Class:** 273 **Joint Degrees Offered:** None. **PharmCAS:** Not required **Minimum GPA:** N/A **Average GPA:** 3.7 **Early Admissions Deadline:** September 1 **Application Deadline:** February 15 **Application Fee:** $30 **In-State Tuition:** $28,400 **Out-of-State Tuition:** $28,400

St. Joseph College School of Pharmacy

229 Trumbull Street, Hartford, CT 06103
Phone: (860) 231-5858
Website: www.sjc.edu/pharmacy
General Info: Saint Joseph College is a private school **Male/Female Ratio:** N/A **Students per Class:** 68 **Joint Degrees Offered:** N/A **PCAT:** Required **PharmCAS:** Required **Minimum GPA:** 2.8 **Average GPA:** N/A **Application Deadline:** March 1 **Application Fee:** $125 **In-State Tuition:** $39,000 **Out-of-State Tuition:** $39,900 **Prerequisites:** English Composition (6 semester hours), Biology I & II w/lab (8 semester hours), Microbiology w/lab (4 semester hours), Human Anatomy & Physiology w/lab (8 semester hours), Physics w/lab (4 semester hours), General Chemistry I & II w/lab (8 semester hours), Organic Chemistry I & II w/lab (8 semester hours), Calculus (3 semester hours), General Economics (3 semester hours), Statistics (3 semester hours), Oral Communication (3 semester hours), Humanities (6 semester hours), Social Science (6 semester hours), Health-related Science (6 semester hours)

Samford University, McWhorter School of Pharmacy

800 Lake Shore Drive, Birmingham, AL 35229
Phone: (205) 726-2820 **Fax:** (205) 726-2759
Website: www.samford.edu/schools/pharmacy. html
General Info: Private school with an acceptance rate of 11.6% to pharmacy school **Pharmacy Student Body:** 478 **Male/Female Ratio:** 30/70 **Students per Class:** 127 **Student/Faculty Ratio:** 14/1 **Joint Degrees Offered:** None **PCAT:** Required. **PharmCAS:** Required. **Minimum GPA:** 2.75 **Average GPA:** 3.55 **Application Deadline:** February 1 **Application Fee:** $50 **In-State Tuition:** $22,280 **Out-of-State Tuition:** $22,280 **Prerequisites:** English Composition (6 semester hours), General Chemistry (8 semester hours), Organic Chemistry (8 semester hours), Anatomy and Physiology (8 semester hours), Precalculus (3 semester hours), Elementary Statistics (3 semester hours), Literature (3 semester hours), Public Speaking (3 semester hours), World History or Western Civilization (3 semester hours), Sociology or Psychology (3 semester hours), Physical Education Activity (2 semester hours), Additional Liberal Arts Electives (9 semester hours).

Shenandoah University Bernard J. Dunn School of Pharmacy

1460 University Drive, Winchester, VA 22601
Phone: (540) 665-1282 **Fax:** (540) 665-1283
Website: www.su.edu/academic/pharmacy.asp
General Info: Private school with an acceptance rate of 6.3% to pharmacy school. **Pharmacy Student Body:** 287 **Male/Female Ratio:** 45/55 **Students per Class:** 75 **Joint Degrees Offered:** PharmD/MBA **PCAT:** Required **Minimum Score:** 60% **PharmCAS:** Required **Minimum GPA:** 2.8 **Average GPA:** 3.5 **Application Deadline:** February 1; rolling admissions. **Application Fee:** $30 **In-State Tuition:** $26,500 **Out-of-State Tuition:** $26,500 **Prerequisites:** English 101 and 102 (6 semester hours), General Chemistry (8 semester hours), Organic Chemistry I and II w/Lab (8 semester hours), General Biology I and II w/Lab, Physics w/Lab (4 semester hours), Microbiology w/Lab (4 semester hours), Math (3 semester hours), Calculus (3 semester hours), Economics (3 semester hours), Biological Elective—no Lab (3 semester hours), Public

Speaking (3 semester hours), Philosophy/
Religion/Ethics or Logic (3 semester hours),
Humanities (3 semester hours), Social/Behavioral
Sciences (6 semester hours).

South Carolina College of Pharmacy

280 Calhoun Street, P.O. Box 250141, Charleston,
SC 29425
Phone: (843) 792-8450 **Fax:** (843) 792-9081
Website: http://sccp.sc.edu/
General Info: Public School with an acceptance
rate of 19.2% to pharmacy school. South Carolina
College of Pharmacy is the merger of the Medical
University of South Carolina College of Pharmacy
in Charleston and the University of South Carolina
College of Pharmacy in Columbia. There is one
application process for admission to both cam-
puses. **Pharmacy Student Body:** 694 **Male/
Female Ratio:** 22/78 **Students per Class:** 202
Joint Degrees Offered: PharmD/PhD, PharmD/
MBA **PCAT:** Required **PharmCAS:** Not required.
Application Deadline: January 1 **Application
Fee:** $75 **In-State Tuition:** $17,647 **Out-of-
State Tuition:** $35,294 **Prerequisites:** General
Chemistry (8 hours), Organic Chemistry (8 hours),
Physics (6 hours), Calculus (3 hours), Statistics
(3 hours), Biology (8 hours), English Composition
(3 hours), English Composition/Literature (3 hours),
Verbal Skills (3 hours), Economics (3 hours),
Psychology (3 hours), Liberal Arts Electives
(9 hours), Human Anatomy/Physiology (6 hours).
Total of 66 hours).

South Dakota State University College of Pharmacy

Box 2202C, 1 Administration Lane, Brookings, SD
57007-0099
Phone: (605) 688-6197 **Fax:** (605) 688-6232
Website: www3.sdstate.edu/academics/colleg-
eofpharmacy/
General Info: Public School with an acceptance
rate of 21.7% to pharmacy school **Pharmacy
Student Body:** 694 **Male/Female Ratio:** 31/69.
Students per Class: 61 **Joint Degrees Offered:**
PharmD/PhD, PharmD/MS **PCAT:** Required
PharmCAS: Not required **Minimum GPA:** 2.5
Average GPA: 3.6 **Application Deadline:** February
1 **In-State Tuition:** $6,542 **Out-of-State Tuition:**
$12,877 **Prerequisites:** General Chemistry w/
Lab, Organic Chemistry w/Lab, General/Cellular

Biology w/Lab, Human Anatomy w/Lab, Human
physiology w/Lab, Microbiology w/Lab, Calculus
I, Economics, English Composition I and II, Public
Speaking, General Education (6 credits from any
of the following areas: Humanities and Arts/
Diversity Electives, Social Sciences/Diversity
Electives, personal wellness).

South University School of Pharmacy – Savannah, GA and Columbia, SC campuses

709 Mall Boulevard, Savannah, GA 31406
Phone: (912) 201-8120 **Fax:** (912) 201-8154
Website: www.southuniversity.edu
General Info: Private school with an acceptance
rate of 12.2% to pharmacy school **Pharmacy
Student Body:** 207. **Male/Female Ratio:** 31/69
Students per Class: 70 **Joint Degrees Offered:**
None. **PCAT:** Required **Minimum Score:** 60%
PharmCAS: Required **Minimum GPA:** 2.80
Average GPA: 3.51 **Early Admissions Deadline:**
September 1 **Application Deadline:** February 1
Application Fee: $50 **In-State Tuition:** $35,180
Out-of-State Tuition: $35,180 **Prerequisites:**
General Chemistry w/Lab (8 semester hours),
Organic Chemistry w/Lab (8 semester hours),
General Biology w/Lab (8 semester hours),
Calculus (3 semester hours), General Physics
w/Lab (8 semester hours), Anatomy and Physiology
w/Lab (8 semester hours), Physics (3 semester
hours), English Composition (3 semester hours),
English Literature (3 semester hours), History
(3 semester hours), Psychology (3 semester hours),
Economics (3 semester hours), Public Speaking
(3 semester hours), Electives (9 semester hours).

Southern Illinois University Edwardsville School of Pharmacy

Campus Box 2000, Edwardsville, IL 62026
Phone: (618) 650-5150 **Fax:** (618) 550-5152
Website: www.siue.edu/pharmacy
General Info: Public school with an acceptance
rate of 20% to pharmacy school **Pharmacy
Student Body:** 82 **Male/Female Ratio:** 48/52
Students per Class: 82 **Joint Degrees Offered:**
None. **PCAT:** Required. **PharmCAS:** Not required
Minimum GPA: 3.0 **Average GPA:** 3.6 **Application
Deadline:** December 1 **Application Fee:** $40
In-State Tuition: $19,665 **Out-of-State Tuition:**
$26,691 **Prerequisites:** English Composition (6

semester hours), Biology w/Lab (8 semester hours), Human Anatomy and Physiology (8 semester hours), General Chemistry w/Lab (10 semester hours), Organic Chemistry w/Lab (8 semester hours), Physics (10 semester hours), Calculus (5 semester hours), Speech/Public Speaking (3 semester hours), Macroeconomics (3 semester hours), Philosophy (3 semester hours), Literature, Music Appreciation, or Art (3 semester hours), Social Sciences (3 semester hours).

Southwestern Oklahoma State University School of Pharmacy

100 Campus Drive, Weatherford, OK 73096
Phone: (580) 774-3760 **Fax:** (580) 774-7020
Website: www.swosu.edu/pharmacy
General Info: Public school with an acceptance rate of 21% to pharmacy school **Pharmacy Student Body:** 326 **Male/Female Ratio:** 44/56 **Students per Class:** 85 Total Faculty: 56 **Student/Faculty Ratio:** 11/1 **Joint Degrees Offered:** None **PCAT:** Required **Minimum Score:** 77% **PharmCAS:** Not required **Minimum GPA:** 2.5 **Average GPA:** 3.5 **Application Deadline:** February 1 **In-State Tuition:** $8,640 **Out-of-State Tuition:** $17,280 **Prerequisites:** Biology I and II w/Lab, Chemistry I and II w/Lab, Calculus, Physics, Organic Chemistry I and II w/Lab, Microbiology. Total of 58 semester hours with a grade of C or better.

St. Louis College of Pharmacy

4588 Parkview Place, St. Louis, MO 63110
Phone: (314) 446-8341 **Fax:** (314) 446-8304
Website: www.stlcop.edu
General Info: Private school with an acceptance rate of 33.3% to pharmacy school. **Pharmacy Student Body:** 1,085 **Male/Female Ratio:** 37/63. **Students per Class:** 179 **Joint Degrees Offered:** PharmD/MS **PCAT:** Not Required **PharmCAS:** Required **Minimum GPA:** 3.50 **Average GPA:** 3.82 **Early Admission Deadline:** December 15 **Application Deadline:** February 1 **Application Fee:** $50 **In-State Tuition:** $22,500 **Out-of-State Tuition:** $22,500 **Prerequisites:** English (6 semester hours), General Chemistry I and II w/Lab (8 semester hours), Organic Chemistry I and II w/Lab (8 semester hours), General Biology w/Lab (5 semester hours), Human Anatomy w/Lab (4 semester hours),

Human Physiology w/Lab (4 semester hours), Calculus I (3 semester hours), Physics I and II (8 semester hours), Introduction to Psychology (3 semester hours), Introduction to Sociology (3 semester hours), Cultural Heritage I and II (6 semester hours), Economics or American Politics (3 semester hours), Literature Elective (3 semester hours).

University at Buffalo, The State University of New York School of Pharmacy and Pharmaceutical Sciences

351 Hochstetter Hall, University at Buffalo, Buffalo, NY 14260-1200
Phone: (716) 645-2825 **Fax:** (716) 645-3688
Website: www.pharmacy.buffalo.edu
General Info: Public school with an acceptance rate of 11.4% to pharmacy school. **Pharmacy Student Body:** 462. **Male/Female Ratio:** 43/57. **Students per Class:** 125. **Student/Faculty Ratio:** 10/1. **Joint Degrees Offered:** PharmD/MBA, PharmD/JD, PharmD/PhD, PharmD/MPH **PCAT:** Required. **PharmCAS:** Not required. **Minimum GPA:** 3.00. **Average GPA:** 3.56. **Early Application Deadline:** November 3. **Application Deadline:** February 2. **Application Fee:** $50. **In-State Tuition:** $8,845. **Out-of-State Tuition:** $14,375. **Prerequisites:** General Chemistry I and II, General Biology I and II w/Lab, Organic Chemistry I and II w/Lab, Calculus I, Physics I and II (Lab optional), Statistics, Economics: micro or macro, Behavioral Sciences (Introduction to Psychology), English Composition I and II, World Civilization I and II, American Pluralism of U.S. History, Arts Elective course.

Sullivan University College of Pharmacy

2100 Gardiner Lane, Louisville, KY 40205
Phone: 502-413-8640
Website: www.sullivan.edu/pharmacy
General Info: Sullivan University is a private school. **Joint Degrees Offered:** None **PCAT required:** Yes **PharmCAS required:** No **Minimum GPA:** 2.5 **Average GPA:** N/A **Application deadline:** December 31 **Application fee:** $100; **In-State Tuition:** $34,000 **Out-of-State Tuition:** $34,000 **Pre-requisites:** General Chemistry w/lab (8 semesters), Organic Chemistry w/lab (8 semesters), General Biology w/lab (8 semesters), Physiology or Anatomy & Physiology

(3 semester hours); Microbiology (4 semesters), Physics (3 semester hours), Calculus (3 semester hours), Statistics (3 semester hours), English Comp. (6 semester hours), General Education (12 semester hours), Economics (3 semester hours)

Temple University School of Pharmacy

3307 N. Broad Street, Philadelphia, PA 19140
Phone: (215) 707-4990; **Fax** (215) 707-3678
Website: www.temple.edu/pharmacy
General Info: Private school with an acceptance rate of 10% to pharmacy school. **Pharmacy Student Body:** 56. **Male/Female Ratio:** 43/57 **Students per Class:** 158 **Joint Degrees Offered:** PharmD/MBA, PharmD/JD **PCAT:** Not required. **PharmCAS:** Required. **Minimum GPA:** N/A. **Average GPA:** 3.5. **Application Deadline:** Rolling admissions. **Application Fee:** $35 **In-State Tuition:** $21,076 **Out-of-State Tuition:** $30,454 **Prerequisites:** English Composition (6 semester hours), General Chemistry I and II (8 semester hours), General Biology I and II (8 semester hours), Organic Chemistry I and II (8 semester hours), Physics I and II (8 semester hours), Calculus I and II (8 semester hours), Macroeconomics (3 semester hours), Intellectual Heritage I and II (6 semester hours), Electives (15 semester hours).

Texas A&M University Health Science Center Irma Lerma Rangel College of Pharmacy

MSC 131, 1010 W. Avenue B, Kingsville, TX 78363-8202
Phone: (361) 593-4272; **Fax:** (361) 593-4233
Website: http://pharmacy.tamhsc.edu
General Info: Public school **Pharmacy Student Body:** 70 **Students per Class:** 87 **Joint Degrees Offered:** None. **PCAT:** Required. **Minimum Score:** 50%. **PharmCAS:** 339 **Minimum GPA:** 2.75. **Average GPA:** Not specified **Application Deadline:** February 1 **Application Fee:** $100 **In-State Tuition:** $30,976 **Out-of-State Tuition:** $37,260. **Prerequisites:** General Chemistry I and II w/Lab (8 semester hours), Organic Chemistry I and II w/Lab (8 semester hours), General Biology I and II w/Lab (8 semester hours), Physics w/Lab (4 semester hours), Molecular Biology/Genetics (3–4 semester hours), Microbiology w/Lab (4 semester hours), Calculus I (3 semester hours), English Composition I and II (6 semester

hours), Communications/Speech (3 semester hours), Electives: Group A courses: Art, Music or Theater (4–6 semester hours), Literature, Philosophy, Language, Anthropology, or Geography (3 semester hours), Sociology, Psychology, Economics, or Computer Science (3 semester hours), History—United States or Texas (6 semester hours), Political Science (6 semester hours). Total of 72–75 semester credit hours needed.

Texas Southern University College of Pharmacy and Health Sciences

3100 Cleburne Street, Houston, TX 77004
Phone: (713) 313-4277 **Fax:** (713) 313-1091
Website: www.tsu.edu
General Info: Public school with an acceptance rate of 16.7% to pharmacy school **Pharmacy Student Body:** 492 **Male/Female Ratio:** 42/58 **Students per Class:** 127 **Joint Degrees Offered:** None. **PCAT:** Required **Minimum Score:** 50%. **PharmCAS:** Not required **Minimum GPA:** 2.00 **Average GPA:** 3.29 **Application Deadline:** February 15 **Application Fee:** $100 **In-State Tuition:** $4,658 **Out-of-State Tuition:** $11,050 **Prerequisites:** General Chemistry I and II w/Lab (8 semester hours), Organic Chemistry I and II w/Lab (8 semester hours), General Biology I and II w/Lab (10 semester hours), Vertebrate Anatomy w/Lab (4 semester hours), Physics w/Lab (4 semester hours), Molecular Biology/Genetics (3–4 semester hours), Microbiology w/Lab (4 semester hours), English Composition I and II (6 semester hours), Literature (3 semester hours), Speech Communications (3 semester hours), Computer Science (3 semester hours), Humanities and Visual Performing Arts (3 semester hours), Political Science: accepted from Texas schools only (6 semester hours). Must earn a C or better in all prepharmacy courses.

Texas Tech University Health Sciences Center School of Pharmacy

1300 Coutler, Suite 112, Amarillo, TX 79106
Phone: (806) 354-5457
Email: pharmacy@ttuhsc.edu
Website: www.ttuhsc.edu
General Info: Public school with an acceptance rate of 16.7% to pharmacy school **Pharmacy Student Body:** 345 **Male/Female Ratio:** 50/50 **Students per Class:** 130; expected to rise to

130 starting with the class of 2011. **Student/ Faculty Ratio:** 6/1 **Joint Degrees Offered:** None. **PCAT:** Required. **Average Composite Score:** 76% **PharmCAS:** Not required. **Minimum GPA:** 3.00. **Average GPA:** 3.67 **Early Admissions Deadline:** January 1 **Application Deadline:** March 1 **Application Fee:** $100 **In-State Tuition:** $10,660 **Out-of-State Tuition:** $22,958 **Prerequisites:** General Chemistry w/Lab (8 semester hours), Organic Chemistry w/Lab (8 semester hours), General Biology w/Lab (8 semester hours), Vertebrate Anatomy w/Lab (4 semester hours), Physics w/Lab (4 semester hours), Microbiology w/Lab (4 semester hours), Calculus (3 semester hours), Statistics (3 semester hours), Speech (3 semester hours), Economics (3 semester hours), English Composition I and II (6 semester hours), English Literature (3 semester hours), Humanities/Social Sciences (15 semester hours minimum).

Thomas J. Long School of Pharmacy and Health Sciences at the University of the Pacific

3601 Pacific Avenue, Stockton, CA 95211
Phone: (209) 946-2561 **Fax:** (209) 946-2410
Website: www.pacific.edu/pharmacy/index.html
General Info: Private school with an acceptance rate of 10% to pharmacy school **Pharmacy Student Body:** 618 **Male/Female Ratio:** 36/64 **Students per Class:** 211 **Joint Degrees Offered:** PharmD/MBA, PharmD/PhD, PharmD/MS **PCAT:** Not required **PharmCAS:** Required **Minimum GPA:** 3.0 **Average GPA:** 3.48 **Application Deadline:** November 1 **Application Fee:** $60 **In-State Tuition:** $52,985 **Out-of-State Tuition:** $52,985 **Prerequisites:** Calculus (3 semester hours), Physics w/Lab (4 semester hours), General Chemistry w/Lab (8 semester hours), Organic Chemistry w/Lab (8 semester hours), General Biology w/Lab (8 semester hours), Microbiology (3 semester hours), English Composition (6 semester hours), Public Speaking (3 semester hours), Psychology (3 semester hours), Macroeconomics (3 semester hours), General Education, Liberal Arts.

Thomas Jefferson University Jefferson School of Pharmacy

130 S. 9th Street, Ste. 1520, Philadelphia, PA 19107
Phone: 215-503-9082
Website: www.jefferson.edu/jchp/pharmacy
General Info: TJU is a private school and has an acceptance rate of 39.5% to its program. **Male/Female Ratio:** 43/57 **Class Size:** 75 **Joint Degrees Offered:** None **PCAT required:** Yes **PharmCAS required:** Yes **Minimum GPA:** 2.7 **Average GPA:** 3.27 **Application deadline:** March 2 **Application fee:** $25 **In-State Tuition:** $28,594 **Out-of-State Tuition:** $28,594 **Pre-requisites:** General Chemistry w/lab (8 semesters), Organic Chemistry w/lab (8 semesters), General Biology w/lab (8 semesters), Physiology or Anatomy & Physiology (8 semesters); Microbiology (4 semesters), Physics (8 semester hours), Calculus (3 semester hours), English Comp. (3 semester hours), Humanities (9 semester hours)

Touro College of Pharmacy (New York)

2090 Adam Clayton Powell Jr. Blvd., Ste. 603, New York, NY 10027
Phone: 212-851-1192
Website: www.touro.edu/pharmacy/
General Information: Touro College of Pharmacy is a private school with an acceptance rate of 36.8% to its pharmacy school. **Male/Female Ratio:** 35/65 **Class Size:** 70 **Joint Degrees Offered:** None **PCAT required:** Yes **PharmCAS required:** Yes **Minimum GPA:** 2.5 **Average GPA:** 3.12 **Application deadline:** February 1 **Application fee:** $55 **In-State Tuition:** $29,680 **Out-of-State Tuition:** $29,680 **Pre-requisites:** General Chemistry w/lab (8 semesters), Organic Chemistry w/lab (8 semesters), General Biology w/lab (8 semesters), Physiology or Anatomy & Physiology (8 semesters); Microbiology (4 semesters), Physics (3 semester hours), Calculus (3 semester hours), Statistics (3 semester hours), Psychology or Sociology (6 semester hours), Speech (3 semester hours), English Comp. (6 semester hours), Economics (3 semester hours), Humanities (6 semester hours); Ethics (3 semester hours)

Touro University–California College of Pharmacy

1310 Johnson Lane, Mare Island, Vallejo, CA 94592
Phone: (707) 638-5221; **Fax:** (707) 638-5266;
Website: http://www.tumi.edu/cop.html
General Info: Private school with an acceptance rate of 9.3% to pharmacy school. **Pharmacy Student Body:** 64. **Male/Female Ratio:** 27/73 **Students per Class:** 100 **Joint Degrees Offered:** None. **PCAT:** Not required **PharmCAS:** Required **Minimum GPA:** 2.75 **Average GPA:** 3.11 **Early Admissions Deadline:** September 1. **Application Deadline:** February 1 **Application Fee:** $50 **In-State Tuition:** $33.000 **Out-of-State Tuition:** $33.000 **Prerequisites:** Calculus (3 semester hours), Inorganic/General Chemistry (8 semester hours), Human Anatomy/Physiology (4 semester hours), Microbiology (4 semester hours), Organic Chemistry (8 hours).

Union University School of Pharmacy

1050 Union University Drive, Jackson, TN 38305
Phone: 731-668-1818
Website: www.uu.edu/academics/sop
General Info: Union University is a private school with an acceptance rate of 40.5% to its pharmacy school. **Male/Female Ratio:** 40/60 **Class Size:** 45 **Joint Degrees Offered:** None **PCAT required:** Yes **PharmCAS required:** Yes **Minimum GPA:** 2.75 **Average GPA:** 3.22 **Application deadline:** March 1 **Application fee:** $50 **In-State Tuition:** $24,150 **Out-of-State Tuition:** $24,150 **Pre-requisites:** General Chemistry w/lab (8 semesters), Organic Chemistry w/lab (8 semesters), General Biology (8 semesters), Physiology or Anatomy & Physiology (8 semesters); Microbiology (3 semesters), Physics (4 semester hours), Calculus (3 semester hours), Biochemistry (6 semester hours), Immunology (6 semester hours) Statistics (3 semester hours), Psychology or Sociology (6 semester hours), Speech (3 semester hours), English Comp. (6 semester hours), Economics (3 semester hours), Humanities (6 semester hours)

University of Arizona College of Pharmacy

Box 210207, Mabel Street, Tucson, AZ 85721
Phone: (520) 626-1427 **Fax:** (520) 626-4063
Website: www.pharmacy.arizona.edu

General Info: Public school with an acceptance rate of 16.7% to pharmacy school **Pharmacy Student Body:** 303 **Male/Female Ratio:** 37/63 **Students per Class:** 82 **Joint Degrees Offered:** PharmD/MBA, PharmD/PhD **PCAT:** Required. **PharmCAS:** Not required **Minimum GPA:** 3.00 **Average GPA:** 3.64 **Application Deadline:** December 1 **Application Fee:** $65 **In-State Tuition:** $15,945 **Out-of-State Tuition:** $30,857 **Prerequisites:** English Composition (6 semester hours), Math (Calculus) (3 semester hours), Humanities (6 semester hours), Behavioral Sciences (6 semester hours), Economics (3 semester hours), Chemistry w/Lab (8 semester hours), Biology w/Lab (8 semester hours), Physics (8 semester hours), Organic Chemistry (8 semester hours), Human Anatomy (8 semester hours), General Microbiology (4).

University of Arkansas for Medical Sciences College of Pharmacy

4301 W. Markham Street, Slot 522, Little Rock, AR 72205
Phone: (501) 686-5557 **Fax:** (501) 686-8315
Website: www.uams.edu/cop
General Info: Public school with an acceptance rate of 50% to pharmacy school. **Pharmacy Student Body:** 380 **Male/Female Ratio:** 37/63 **Student/Faculty Ratio:** 6/1 **Full-Time Faculty:** 62 **Joint Degrees Offered:** PharmD/MPH, PharmD/MBA Nuclear Pharmacy Option: Recently, the school of pharmacy expanded its program and now offers a program geared for nuclear pharmacy. The program meets the requirements of the Nuclear Regulatory Commission (NCR). Students can train in this area through internships or following graduation. To learn more, visit the website above. **PCAT:** Required; incoming students rank within the 77th percentile **PharmCAS:** Not required **Minimum GPA:** 2.00 **Average GPA:** 3.48 **Application Deadline:** February 1 **Application Fee:** $60 **In-State Tuition:** $8,400 **Out-of-State Tuition:** $16,800 **Prerequisites:** Core courses: Math (3–5 semester hours to include Calculus I), Chemistry (16 semester hours to include College Chemistry I and II w/Lab and Organic Chemistry I and II w/Lab), Biology (12 semester hours to include General Biology I and II w/Lab and Microbiology w/Lab), Physics (4 semester hours to include General Physics w/Lab), Non-Core

Courses: English/Communications (9 semester hours), Economics/Accounting (3 semester hours), Humanities Electives (69 semester hours).

University of California–San Diego Skaggs School of Pharmacy

9500 Gilman Drive, La Jolla, CA 92093-0657
Phone: (858) 822-4900 **Fax:** (858) 534-8248
Website: www.ucsd.edu
General Info: Public school with an acceptance rate of 5.6% to pharmacy school **Pharmacy Student Body:** 140 **Male/Female Ratio:** 27/73 **Students per Class:** 60 **Joint Degrees Offered:** PharmD/MBA **PCAT:** Not required **PharmCAS:** Required **Minimum GPA:** 3.00 **Average GPA:** 3.67 **Application Deadline:** November 1 **Application Fee:** $50 **In-State Tuition:** $7,596 **Out-of-State Tuition:** $11,678 **Prerequisites:** English w/Writing Component (6 semester hours), General Chemistry w/Lab (8 semester hours), Organic Chemistry w/Lab (8 semester hours), Biology: cellular, molecular ,and whole animal (8 semester hours), Physics w/Labs in Electricity and Magnetism (6 semester hours), Calculus w/Analytical Geometry (6 semester hours), Economics (3 semester hours), Public Speaking or Debate (3 semester hours), Human Behavior (3 semester hours), Electives (12 semester hours).

University of California–San Francisco

513 Pamassus Avenue, 0150, Room S-960, San Francisco, CA 94143
Phone: (415) 476-2732 **Fax:** (415) 476-6805
Website: http://pharmacy.ucsf.edu/pharmd/
General Info: Public school with an acceptance rate of 8.7% to pharmacy school. **Pharmacy Student Body:** 490 **Male/Female Ratio:** 25/75 **Student/Faculty Ratio:** 11/1 **Students per Class:** 122 **Joint Degrees Offered:** PharmD/MPH, PharmD/PhD **Unique "Pathways":** options in degree emphasis: Pharmaceutical Care, Pharmaceutical Health Policy and Management, Pharmaceutical Sciences **PCAT:** Not required **PharmCAS:** Required. **Minimum GPA:** 2.80 **Average GPA:** 3.58 **Application Deadline:** November 1 **Application Fee:** $60 (US citizen), $80 (non-U.S. citizen) **In-State Tuition:** $18,240 **Out-of-State Tuition:** $30,485 **Prerequisites:**

General Chemistry w/Lab (minimum 12 quarter units), Organic Chemistry w/Lab (minimum 12 quarter units), General Biology (minimum 12 quarter units), Physiology (minimum 4 quarter units), Physics w/ELM Lab (minimum 8 quarter units), Calculus (minimum 8 quarter units), English Composition (minimum 8 quarter units), Economics: Micro or Macro (minimum 4 quarter units), Public Speaking (minimum 4 quarter units), Cultural Anthropology, Psychology or Sociology (minimum 4 quarter units).

University of Charleston School of Pharmacy

2300 MacCorkle Avenue, SE, Charleston, WV 25304
Phone: 304-357-4858 **Fax:** 304-357-4868
Website: www.ucwv.edu/academics/pharmacy
General Info: Private school **Male/Female Ratio:** 45/55 **Student/Faculty Ratio:** 10/1 **Students per Class:** 75 **Joint Degrees Offered:** None **PCAT:** Required **PharmCAS:** Required **Minimum GPA:** 2.75 **Average GPA:** 3.40 **Early Admissions:** Not offered **Application Deadline:** February 1 **Application fee:** $50 **In-State Tuition:** $24,080 **Out-of-State Tuition:** $24,080 **Prerequisites:** Human Anatomy and Physiology (8 semester hours), General biology w/lab (8 semester hours), General Chemistry w/lab (8 semester hours), Microbiology w/lab (4 semester hours), Organic Chemistry w/lab (8 semester hours), Physics w/lab (4 semester hours), Statistics (2 semester hours), Algebra (3 semester hours), Calculus (3 semester hours), Ethics (3 semester hours), Economics (3 semester hours), English Composition (6 semester hours), Psychology or Sociology (3 semester hours), History or Political Science (3 semester hours)

University of Cincinnati James L. Winkle College of Pharmacy

P.O. Box 670004, Cincinnati, OH 45267-0004
Phone: (513) 558-3326 **Fax:** (513) 558-4372
Website: www.pharmacy.uc.edu
General Info: Public school with an acceptance rate of 16.7% to pharmacy school **Pharmacy Student Body:** 309 **Male/Female Ratio:** 45/55 **Students per Class:** 96 **Joint Degrees Offered:** None. **PCAT:** Required **PharmCAS:** Required **Minimum GPA:** 2.85 **Average GPA:** 3.50 **Application Deadline:** December 31 **Application**

Fee: Not available **In-State Tuition:** $9,399 **Out-of-State Tuition:** $23,922 **Prerequisites:** English Composition (9 semester hours), Math (Calculus) (9 semester hours), Chemistry w/Lab (15 semester hours), Biology w/Lab (15 semester hours), Physics (15 semester hours), Statistics (3 semester hours), Microbiology (3 semester hours).

University of Colorado–Denver School of Pharmacy

12631 E. 17th Avenue, Aurora, CO 80045
Phone: (303) 724-1234 **Fax:** (303) 724-2627
Website: www.ucdenver.edu/pharmacy
General Info: Public school with an acceptance rate of 11.1% to pharmacy school **Pharmacy Student Body:** 515 **Male/Female Ratio:** 35/65 **Students per Class:** 136 **Joint Degrees Offered:** None **PCAT:** Not required **PharmCAS:** Required **Minimum GPA:** 3.00 **Average GPA:** 3.46 **Application Deadline:** December 1 **Application Fee:** $50 **In-State Tuition:** $17,928 **Out-of-State Tuition:** $29,982 **Prerequisites:** General Chemistry w/Lab (8 semester hours), Organic Chemistry w/Lab (8 semester hours), General Biology w/Lab (8 semester hours), Microbiology w/Lab (4 semester hours), Human Anatomy or Human Anatomy and Physiology (3–4 semester hours), General Physics (3 semester hours), Calculus I (3 semester hours), English Composition (6 semester hours), Social Sciences (3 semester hours), Microeconomics (3 semester hours), Public Speaking (3 semester hours), General Education: no vocational, technical, or physical education courses. All courses must be completed with a C or better; C- is not acceptable.

University of Connecticut School of Pharmacy

69 N. Eagleville Road, Unit 3092, Storrs, CT 06269-3092
Phone: (860) 486-2129 **Fax:** (860) 486-1553
Website: http://pharmacy.uconn.edu
General Info: Public school with an acceptance rate of 21.7% to pharmacy school **Pharmacy Student Body:** 390 **Male/Female Ratio:** 42/58 **Students per Class:** 102 **Joint Degrees Offered:** None **PCAT:** Yes **PharmCAS:** Not required **Minimum GPA:** 3.0 **Average GPA:** 3.30.

Application Deadline: February 1 **Application Fee:** Not available. **In-State Tuition:** $6,456 **Out-of-State Tuition:** $19,656 **Prerequisites:** English Composition (4 semester hours), Math (Calculus) (4 semester hours), Chemistry w/Lab (8 semester hours), Biology w/Lab (4 semester hours), Physics (3 semester hours), Organic Chemistry (6 semester hours), Microeconomics (3 semester hours), Anatomy (6 semester hours), Microbiology (4 semester hours), Biochemistry (4 semester hours), Sociology (3 semester hours), Electives (15 semester hours).

University of Findlay College of Pharmacy

1000 N. Main Street, Findlay, OH 45840
Phone: (419) 434-5327 **Fax:** (419) 434-697
Website: www.findlay.edu
General Info: Private school, 6-year degree program. **Pharmacy Student Body:** Not available. **Male/Female Ratio:** Not available **Students per Class:** Not available **Joint Degrees Offered:** None **PCAT:** Not required **PharmCAS:** Not required **Minimum GPA:** N/A **Average GPA:** Not available **Application Deadline:** February 1 **Application Fee:** $50 **In-State Tuition:** $26,836 **Out-of-State Tuition:** $26,836 **Prerequisites:** Fine arts (3 semester hours), Humanities (3 semester hours), Social Sciences (3 semester hours), Foreign Language (3 semester hours), Natural Sciences (3 semester hours), Mathematics (3 semester hours), English (3 semester hours), Philosophy or Religion (3 semester hours).

University of Florida College of Pharmacy

Box 100484, J. Hillis Miller Health Center, Gainesville, FL 32610
Phone: (352) 392-9714 **Fax:** (352) 392-3480
Website: www.cop.ufl.edu
General Info: Public school with an acceptance rate of 16.1% to pharmacy school. (10% out of state) **Pharmacy Student Body:** 1,147 **Male/Female Ratio:** 39/61 **Students per Class:** 180 **Joint Degrees Offered:** PharmD/MBA, PharmD/MPH, PharmD/JD, PharmD/PhD **PCAT:** Required **PharmCAS:** Required **Minimum GPA:** 3.00 **Average GPA:** 3.48 **Application Deadline:** February 1 **Application Fee:** $30 **In-State Tuition:** $14,503 **Out-of-State Tuition:** $14,503 **Prerequisites:** Math (Calculus) (3 semester hours), Chemistry w/Lab (8 semester hours),

Biology w/Lab (8 semester hours), Physics (8 semester hours), Organic Chemistry (8 semester hours), Public Speaking (3 semester hours), Anatomy and Physiology (8 semster hours).

University of Georgia College of Pharmacy

RC Wilson Building, University of Georgia, Athens, GA 30602-2351
Phone: (706) 542-1914 **Fax:** (706) 542-5269
Website: www.rx.uga.edu
General Info: Public school with an acceptance rate of 13.7% to pharmacy school **Pharmacy Student Body:** 496 **Male/Female Ratio:** 44/56 **Students per Class:** 132 **Joint Degrees Offered:** None. **PCAT:** Required. **Minimum Score:** none **PharmCAS:** Not required **Minimum GPA:** N/A **Average GPA:** 3.54 **Early Admissions Deadline:** September 1 **Application Deadline:** February 1 **Application Fee:** $55 **In-State Tuition:** $6,338 **Out-of-State Tuition:** $15,345 **Prerequisites:** English (6 semester hours), Math (Precalculus) (3 semester hours), Calculus (4 semester hours), Economics (3 semester hours), Political Science (American Government) (3 semester hours), History (3 semester hours), Communications (Public Speaking and Interpersonal Communication) (6 semester hours), Chemistry I and II (8 semester hours), Organic Chemistry (8 semester hours), Biology I and II (8 semester hours), Statistics (4 semester hours).

University of Hawaii Hilo College of Pharmacy

60 Nowelo St. ste. 101, Hilo, HI 96720
Phone: 808-443-5900, **Email:** pharmacy@hawaii.edu; **Website:** http://pharmacy.uhh.hawaii.edu/
General Info: The University of HI college of pharmacy is a new program. Matriculation for this college began in 2007. A lot of statistical information has yet to be determined. To learn about the most recent statistical information, to include average GPA, contact the school (email listed above) **Class Enrollment:** 90 **Joint Degrees Offered:** None **PCAT:** Required **PharmCAS:** Required. **Minimum GPA:** none **Average GPA:** TBD **Early Admissions:** Not offered **Application Deadline:** November 1 **Application fee:** $50 **In-State Tuition:** $8,269 **Out-of-State Tuition:** $16,537 **Prerequisites:** Human Anatomy/Physiology (8 semester hours), Biology w/lab

(8 semester hrs), Microbiology w/lab (4 semester hours), General Chemistry w/lab (8 semester hours), Quantitative Reasoning/Math/Calculus (3 semester hours), English Composition (6 semester hours), World Cultures (3 semester hours), Humanities (9 semester hours), Social Behavioral Sciences (3 semester hours), Economics (3 semester hours), Speech (3 semester hours)

University of Houston College of Pharmacy

141 Sciences and Research Building 2, 4800 Calhoun, Houston, TX 77294
Phone: (713) 743-1239 **Fax:** (713) 743-5678
Website: www.uh.edu/pharmacy
General Info: Public School with an acceptance rate of 16.4% to pharmacy school. **Pharmacy Student Body:** 485 **Male/Female Ratio:** 36/66 **Students per Class:** 125 **Joint Degrees Offered:** PharmD/PhD, PharmD/MS in pharmacy administration **PCAT:** Required **Minimum Score:** 83.6% **PharmCAS:** Not required **Minimum GPA:** 2.70 **Average GPA:** 3.56 **Application Deadline:** February 15 **Application Fee:** $100 **In-State Tuition:** $13,660 **Out-of-State Tuition:** $22,096 **Prerequisites:** Biology w/Lab (8 semester hours), Chemistry w/Lab (8 semester hours), English (6 semester hours), U.S. History (6 semester hours), Calculus (3 semester hours), Statistics (3 semester hours), Humanities (3 semester hours), Organic Chemistry w/Lab (10 semester hours), Political Science (3 semester hours), Social Science (Intro to Psychology or Sociology and Writing Intensive Course) (6 semester hours), Physics (3 semester hours), Visual Arts (3 semester hours), Microbiology w/Lab (4 semester hours), Communication/Speech (3 semester hours).

University of Illinois–Chicago College of Pharmacy

833 S. Wood Street, M/C 874, Chicago, IL 60612
Phone: (312) 996-7242 **Fax:** (312) 966-3272
Website: www.uic.edu/pharmacy
General Info: Public school with an acceptance rate of 11% to pharmacy school **Pharmacy Student Body:** 650 **Male/Female Ratio:** 31/69 **Students per Class:** 162 **Joint Degrees Offered:** PharmD/PhD, PharmD/MBA, PharmD/MSHI. **PCAT:** Required **PharmCAS:** Required **Minimum GPA:** 2.50 **Average GPA:** 3.31 **Application**

Deadline: December 1 **Application Fee:** $40 (U.S. citizen); $50 (international applicants). **In-State Tuition:** $13,708 **Out-of-State Tuition:** $21,120 **Prerequisites:** English (6 semester hours), Speech/Communication (2 semester hours), General Biology w/Lab (8 semester hours), General Chemistry w/Lab (8 semester hours), Organic Chemistry w/Lab (8 semester hours), Physics w/Lab (8 semester hours), Calculus (3 semester hours), Human Anatomy (4 semester hours), General Education: Social/Behavioral Sciences (3 semester hours), Economics (3 semester hours), Humanities (3 semester hours). Total pre-pharmacy coursework 60 semester hours.

University of the Incarnate Word Feik School of Pharmacy

4301 Broadway, CPO #99, San Antonio, TX 78209 **Phone:** (210) 805-3012 **Fax:** (210) 805-3013 **Website:** http://www.uiw.edu/pharmacy **General Info:** Private school. **Pharmacy Student Body:** 80 **Male/Female Ratio:** Not reported **Students per Class:** 80 **Joint Degrees Offered:** None. **PCAT:** Required **PharmCAS:** Not required **Minimum GPA:** 2.5 **Average GPA:** Not specified **Application Deadline:** January 5 **Application Fee:** $100. **In-State Tuition:** $25,500 **Out-of-State Tuition:** $25,500 **Prerequisites:** General Chemistry I and II w/Lab (8 semester hours), Precalculus (3 semester hours), Calculus (3 semester hours), Biology I (4 semester hours), Physical Education (1 semester hour), English Composition I and II (6 semester hours), Introduction to Philosophy (3 semester hours), Organic Chemistry I and II w/Lab (8 semester hours), Physics I w/Lab (4 semester hours), Human Physiology (4 semester hours), World Literature Studies (3 semester hours), Fine Arts (3 semester hours), Social Sciences (3 semester hours), Religion (3 semester hours), Introduction to Probability and Statistics (3 semester hours), History (3 semester hours).

University of Iowa College of Pharmacy

115 S. Grand Avenue, Iowa City, IA 52242 **Phone:** (319) 335-8795 **Fax:** (319) 335-5594 **Website:** http://pharmacy.uiowa.edu **General Info:** Public school with an acceptance rate of 14.3% to pharmacy school. **Pharmacy**

Student Body: 428 **Male/Female Ratio:** 41/59 **Students per Class:** 110 **Joint Degrees Offered:** PharmD/MBA **PCAT:** Required **PharmCAS:** Required **Minimum GPA:** 2.50 **Average GPA:** 3.52 **Application Deadline:** December 1 **Application Fee:** $100 **In-State Tuition:** $17,263 per semester **Out-of-State Tuition:** $9,535 per semester **Prerequisites:** English composition (4+ semester hours), General Chemistry I and II w/Lab (8 semester hours), Organic Chemistry I and II (6 semester hours), Biology I and II (8 semester hours), Anatomy (3 semester hours), Microbiology (4 semester hours), Calculus for Biological Sciences (4 semester hours), Physiology (4 semester hours), Physics (4 semester hours), Microeconomics (4 semester hours), Statistics (3 semester hours), General Education Electives (12 semester hours).

University of Kansas School of Pharmacy

1251 Wesco Hall Drive, Room 2056 Malott Hall, Lawrence, KS 66045 **Phone:** (785) 864-3591 **Fax:** (785) 864-5265 **Website:** www.pharm.ku.edu **General Info:** Public school with an acceptance rate of 22.2% to pharmacy school **Pharmacy Student Body:** 414 **Male/Female Ratio:** 42/58 **Students per Class:** 105 **Joint Degrees Offered:** PharmD/MBA **PCAT:** Required **PharmCAS:** Not required. **Minimum GPA:** N/A **Average GPA:** 3.57 **Application Deadline:** February 1. **Application Fee:** $50. **In-State Tuition:** $2,295 per semester. **Out-of-State Tuition:** $5,485 per semester. **Prerequisites:** English Composition (6 semester hours), General Chemistry I and II w/Lab (10 semester hours), Organic Chemistry I and II w/Lab (10 semester hours), Molecular and Cellular Biology (4 semester hours), Anatomy (3 semester hours), Microbiology (4 semester hours), Calculus (3 semester hours), Physiology w/Lab (6 semester hours), Physics (4 semester hours), General Education Electives (18 semester hours).

University of Kentucky College of Pharmacy

725 Rose St., Suite 237, Lexington, KY 40536-0082 **Phone:** (859) 323-7601; **Fax:** (859) 257-2128; **Website:** www.uky.edu/pharmacy **General Info:** Public school with an acceptance rate of 15.7% to pharmacy school **Pharmacy**

Student Body: 453 **Male/Female Ratio:** 37/63 **Student/Faculty Ratio:** 7/1 **Students per Class:** 132. **Joint Degrees Offered:** PharmD/MPA, PharmD/PhD, PharmD/MBA, PharmD/MS in economics **PCAT:** Required **Minimum Score:** 50%. **PharmCAS:** Required **Minimum GPA:** 2.50 **Average GPA:** 3.25 **Early Admissions Deadline:** September 3 **Application Deadline:** January 15 **Application Fee:** $75 **In-State Tuition:** $19,376 **Out-of-State Tuition:** $35,270 **Prerequisites:** English (6–7 semester hours), Animal Biology w/Lab (4–5 semester hours), Microbiology w/Lab (4–5 semester hours), Calculus (4 semester hours; can bypass calculus by taking both college Algebra and Elementary Calculus, 6 semester hours), Statistics (3 semester hours), Human Anatomy or Physiology (3 semester hours) (Non-University of Kentucky students can take Physiology or combined AP courses if Anatomy is not offered at school), General Chemistry w/Lab (8–10 semester hours), Organic Chemistry w/Lab (8–10 semester hours), Physics w/Lab (8–10 semester hours; if the physics lecture courses are a minimum of 8 hours then labs are not needed), Microeconomics (3 semester hours), Elective Courses (10–20 semester hours).

University of Louisiana–Monroe College of Pharmacy

700 University Avenue, Monroe, LA 1209-0400
Phone: (318) 342-1600 **Fax:** (318) 342-1606
Website: www.ulm.edu
General Info: Public school with an acceptance rate of 20% to pharmacy school **Pharmacy Student Body:** 429 **Male/Female Ratio:** 34/66 **Students per Class:** 98 **Joint Degrees Offered:** None. **PCAT:** Required **PharmCAS:** Required. **Minimum GPA:** 3.00 **Average GPA:** 3.71 **Application Deadline:** March 2. **Application Fee:** $75 **In-State Tuition:** $4,618 **Out-of-State Tuition:** $9,952 **Prerequisites:** English Composition (6 semester hours), General Chemistry I and II w/Lab (8 semester hours), Organic Chemistry I and II w/Lab (8 semester hours), Biology (8 semester hours), Kinesiology (1 semester hour), Social Sciences (3 semester hours), Fine Arts (3 semester hours), Humanities Electives (9 semester hours), Calculus (6 semester hours), Physics (6 semester hours), Psychology (3 semester hours), Accounting (3 semester hours), Economics (3 semester hours).

University of Maryland Eastern Shore School of Pharmacy

Somerset Hall, Room 116, Princess Anne, MD 21853
Phone: (410) 621-2292
Website: www.umes.edu/pharmacy
General Info: University of Maryland Eastern Shore is a public school **Male/Female Ratio:** 50/50 **Students per Class:** 60 **Joint Degrees Offered:** N/A **PCAT:** Required **PharmCAS:** Required **Minimum GPA:** 2.75 **Average GPA:** 3.3 **Application Deadline:** February 1 **Application Fee:** $25 **In-State Tuition:** $39,000 **Out-of-State Tuition:** $39,900 **Prerequisites:** English Composition and/or Literature (6 semester hours); Biology w/lab (4 semester hours), Microbiology w/lab (4 semester hours), Anatomy & Physiology w/lab (8 semester hours), Physics w/lab (4 semester hours), General Chemistry w/lab (8 semester hours), Organic Chemistry w/lab (8 semester hours), Calculus (4 semester hours), Statistics (3 semester hours), General Economics (3 semester hours), Public Speaking (3 semester hours), Art & Humanities/Social & Behavioral Sciences (12 semester hours)

University of Maryland School of Pharmacy

20 N. Pine Street, Room 730, Baltimore, MD 21201-1180
Phone: (410) 706-7651 **Fax:** (410) 706-4012
Website: www.pharmacy.umaryland.edu
General Info: Public school with an acceptance rate of 7.7% to pharmacy school **Pharmacy Student Body:** 489 **Male/Female Ratio:** 42/58 **Students per Class:** 124 **Joint Degrees Offered:** PharmD/JD, PharmD/PhD, PharmD/MBA, PharmD/MPH **PCAT:** Required. **Minimum Score:** 80% **PharmCAS:** Not required. **Minimum GPA:** 2.5 **Average GPA:** 3.4 **Early Admissions Deadline:** September 1 **Application Deadline:** January 5 **Application Fee:** $30 **In-State Tuition:** $12,637 **Out-of-State Tuition:** $26,122 **Prerequisites:** English Composition (3 semester hours), Calculus (3 semester hours), Statistics (3 semester hours), Biology w/Lab (4 semester hours), Microbiology w/Lab (4 semester hours), General Chemistry w/Lab (8 semester hours), Organic Chemistry w/Lab (8 semester hours), Physics (8 semester hours), Human Anatomy and Physiology (6 semester hours), Humanities and Social Sciences (18 semester hours), Speech

Communication (1 course), Microeconomics or Macro-/Microeconomics (1 course).

University of Michigan College of Pharmacy

428 Church Street, Ann Arbor, MI 48109-1065
Phone: (734) 764-7144 **Fax:** (734) 763-2022
Website: www.umich.edu/~pharmacy/
General Info: Public school with an acceptance rate of 33.3% to pharmacy school. **Pharmacy Student Body:** 267 **Male/Female Ratio:** 42/58 **Students per Class:** 73 **Joint Degrees Offered:** PharmD/PhD, PharmD/MS **PCAT:** Required **PharmCAS:** Not required **Minimum GPA:** None specified **Average GPA:** 3.40 **Application Deadline:** February 1 **Application Fee:** $40 (U.S. citizen); $55 (international applicants). **In-State Tuition:** $17,578 **Out-of-State Tuition:** $32,368 **Prerequisites:** General Biology (2 semester), General Chemistry w/Lab (2 semesters), Organic Chemistry w/Lab (2 semesters), Physics (2 semesters), English Composition and Literature (1 semester), Calculus (1 semester), Genetics (1 semester), Social Science (2 semesters), Medical Microbiology w/Lab (1 semester), Human Anatomy (1 semester), General Statistics (3 semesters), Humanities and/or foreign languages (2 semesters).

University of Minnesota College of Pharmacy

308 Harvard Street, 5-130 Weaver-Densford Hall, Minneapolis, MN 55-455-0343
Phone: (612) 624-1900 **Fax:** (612) 915-5118
Website: www.pharmacy.umn.edu
General Info: Public school with an acceptance rate of 17.9% to pharmacy school **Pharmacy Student Body:** 583 **Male/Female Ratio:** 35/65 **Students per Class:** 161 **Joint Degrees Offered:** PharmD/PhD **PCAT:** Required **PharmCAS:** Required. **Minimum GPA:** 3.00 **Average GPA:** 3.57 **Early Admissions Deadline:** September 1 **Application Deadline:** February 17 **Application Fee:** $75 **In-State Tuition:** $17,126 **Out-of-State Tuition:** $28,564 **Prerequisites:** General Biology w/Lab (2 courses), Microbiology w/Lab (1 course), Human Anatomy and/or Human Anatomy and Physiology w/Lab (1 course), General Chemistry w/Lab (sufficient to qualify for organic chemistry), Organic Chemistry w/Lab (entire sequence), General Physics w/Labs (entire introductory sequence, courses dealing with human

behavior in society—psychology or sociology courses; 2 courses), Calculus (1 course), English Composition (2 courses), Economics (1 course), Public Speaking (1 course), Statistics.

University of Mississippi School of Pharmacy

P.O. Box 1848, University, MS 38377
Phone: (662) 915-7265 **Fax:** (662) 915-5118
Website: www.olemiss.edu/depts/pharm_school
General Info: Public school with an acceptance rate of 17.9% to pharmacy school **Pharmacy Student Body:** 428 **Male/Female Ratio:** 31/69 **Students per Class:** 83 **Joint Degrees Offered:** PharmD/PhD **PCAT:** Required **PharmCAS:** Not required **Minimum GPA:** 2.75 **Average GPA:** 3.68. **Application Deadline:** February 1 **In-State Tuition:** $8,154 **Out-of-State Tuition:** $14,622 **Prerequisites:** English (6 semester hours), General Chemistry I and II (8 semester hours), Biology I and II (8 semester hours), Organic Chemistry I and II (8 semester hours), Physics I and II (8 semester hours), Calculus (3 semester hours), Statistics (3 semester hours), Speech (3 semester hours), Microeconomics (3 semester hours), Electives (15 semester hours), Bio Medethics, Bio Chemistry, Genetics.

University of Missouri-Kansas City School of Pharmacy

5100 Rockhill Road, Kansas City, MO 64110-2499
Phone: 816-235-1609. **Fax:** 816-235-5190.
Website: www.umkc.edu/pharmacy
General Info: Public school with an acceptance rate of 20% to pharmacy school. **Pharmacy Student Body:** 484. **Male/Female Ratio:** 34/66 **Students per Class:** 77 **Joint Degrees Offered:** PharmD/MBA. **PCAT:** Required **PharmCAS:** No. **Minimum GPA:** 2.75 **Average GPA:** 3.54 **Application Deadline:** December 15 **Application Fee:** $35 (US citizen); $50 (international applicants). **In-State Tuition:** $17,146 **Out-of-State Tuition:** $36,616 **Prerequisites:** General chemistry I&II w/labs (8 semester hours), Calculus (4 semester hours), General biology I & II (6 semester hours), Physics w/lab (4 semester hours), English Composition I & II (6 semester hours), Behavioral/Social Sciences &/or Humanities/Fine Arts electives (3 semester hours)

University of Montana College of Health Professionals and Biomedical Sciences, Skaggs School of Pharmacy

3450 Skaggs Building, Missoula, MT 59812-1512
Phone: (406) 243-4656; **Fax:** (406) 243-4209.
Website: www.health.umt.edu
General Info: Public school with an acceptance rate of 22% to pharmacy school **Pharmacy Student Body:** 254 **Male/Female Ratio:** 41/59 **Student/Faculty Ratio:** 6/1 **Students per Class:** 65 **Full-Time Faculty Members:** 42 **Joint Degrees Offered:** PharmD/PhD, PharmD/MBA **PCAT:** Required. Students should rank within the 78th percentile. **PharmCAS:** Not required **Minimum GPA:** 2.5 **Average GPA:** 3.5 **Application Deadline:** February 15 **Application Fee:** $50 **In-State Tuition:** $10,692 **Out-of-State Tuition:** $24,024 **Prerequisites:** First Year: College Chemistry (6 semester credits), College Chemistry Lab (4 semester credits), Social Science Elective (Psychology or Sociology) (3 semester credits), Applied Calculus (3 semester credits), English Composition (3 semester credits), Intro to Micro or Macro Economics (3 semester credits), Electives and General Education (9 semester credits). Second Year: Organic Chemistry (6 semester credits), Organic Chemistry w/Lab (4 semester credits), Communications Elective (3 semester credits), Cellular and Molecular Biology (4 semester credits), College Physics w/Lab (5 semester hours), Statistics (4 semester hours), Electives and General Education (8 semester hours). All prerequisites must be completed with a C or better.

University of Nebraska Medical Center College of Pharmacy

986000 Nebraska Medical Center, Omaha, NE 68198-6000
Phone: (402) 559-4333 **Fax:** (402) 559-5060
Website: www.unmc.edu/pharmacy
General Info: Public school with an acceptance rate of 23.8% to pharmacy school. **Pharmacy Student Body:** 259 **Male/Female Ratio:** 28/72 **Students per Class:** 65 **Joint Degrees Offered:** PharmD/MS, PharmD/MBA, PharmD/PhD **PCAT:** Not required **PharmCAS:** Not required **Minimum GPA:** 3.0 **Average GPA:** 3.72 **Application Deadline:** January 1 **Application Fee:** $45 **In-State Tuition:** $15,230 **Out-of-State Tuition:**

$22,290 **Prerequisites:** Chemical and Biological Sciences (minimum of 24 semester hours): General Chemistry w/Lab (8 semester hours), Organic Chemistry w/Lab (8 semester hours), Biological/Life Sciences w/Lab (8 semester hours). English Composition I (3 semester hours), English Composition II or Speech (3 semester hours). Calculus (3–5 semester hours), Statistics or Biostatistics (3 semester hours), Quantitative Chemical Analysis or Physics (4–8 semester hours). Accounting (3 semester hours), Economics (3 semester hours). Psychology (3 semester hours), Advanced Psychology or Sociology or Gerontology (3 semester hours), Molecular Biology (3 semester hours), Anatomy (4 semester hours), Physiology (4 semester hours).Choose at least two courses from the following and/or related areas: Humanities, Ethics, Political Science, Foreign Languages, Business Administration, History, Logic, Literature, Fine Arts, Critical Thinking, Philosophy.

University of New England College of Pharmacy

716 Stevens Avenue, Portland, ME 04103
Phone: (207) 221-4225
Website: www.une.edu/pharmacy
General Info: University of New England is a public school **Male/Female Ratio:** N/A **Students per Class:** 100 **Joint Degrees Offered:** N/A **PCAT:** Required **PharmCAS:** Required **Minimum GPA:** 2.5 **Average GPA:** 3.3 **Application Deadline:** February 1 **Application Fee:** $0 **In-State Tuition:** $30,990 **Out-of-State Tuition:** $30,990 **Prerequisites:** English Composition (6 semester hours), Biology I/II w/lab (8 semester hours), Anatomy & Physiology I/II w/lab (8 semester hours), Physics w/lab (4 semester hours), General Chemistry I/II w/lab (8 semester hours), Organic Chemistry I/II w/lab (8 semester hours), Calculus (4 semester hours), Statistics (3 semester hours), Psychology (3 semester hours), Public Speaking (3 semester hours), Human Behavior/Social Sciences (3 semester hours), General Education/Liberal Arts Electives (12 semester hours)

University of New Mexico College of Pharmacy

MSCO9-5360, 1 University of New Mexico, Albuquerque, NM 87131-5691
Phone: (502) 272-0906 **Fax:** (502) 272-6749
Website: http://hsc.unm.edu/pharmacy
General Info: Public school with an acceptance rate of 6.4% to pharmacy school. **Pharmacy Student Body:** 1,331 **Male/Female Ratio:** 35/65 **Students per Class:** 85 Total Faculty Members: 45 **Joint Degrees Offered:** None **PCAT:** Required **Minimum Score:** 30%. **PharmCAS:** Required **Minimum GPA:** 2.5 **Average GPA:** 3.5 **Early Admissions Deadline:** September 1 **Application Deadline:** February 1 **Application Fee:** $40 **In-State Tuition:** $506.35 per credit. **Out-of-State Tuition:** $1,183 per credit. **Prerequisites:** General Biology I w/Lab (4 semester hours), General Chemistry I and II w/Lab (8 semester hours), Organic Chemistry I and II w/Lab (8 semester hours), General Physics (3 semester hours), Calculus I (3 semester hours), Microbiology w/Lab (4 semester hours), Human Anatomy and Physiology I and II (8 semester hours), Statistics (3 semester hours), Microeconomics (3 semester hours), Communications Selective (3 semester hours), Critical Thinking Selective (3 semester hours), Electives (6 semester hours).

University of North Carolina at Chapel Hill Eshelman School of Pharmacy.

Beard Hall, CB #7360, Chapel Hill, NC 27599-7360
Phone: (919) 966-9429 **Fax:** (919) 966-6919
Website: www.pharmacy.unc.edu
General Info: Public school with an acceptance rate of 25% to pharmacy school. **Pharmacy Student Body:** 515 **Male/Female Ratio:** 35/65. **Students per Class:** 152 **PCAT:** Required **PharmCAS:** Required **Minimum GPA:** 2.8 **Average GPA:** 3.5 **Application Deadline:** November 1 **Application Fee:** $73 **In-State Tuition:** $14,877 **Out-of-State Tuition:** $32,803 **Prerequisites:** General Chemistry I (4 semester hours), Organic Chemistry I and II w/Lab (7–8 semester hours), Biology I (4 semester hours), Biology: Human Anatomy and Physiology (4 semester hours), Microbiology (4 semester hours), Physics I and II (8 semester hours), Calculus (3 semester hours), Statistics (3 semester hours), Foreign Language (9–10 semester hours), Social and Behavioral Sciences (9 semester hours), Humanities and Fine Arts (9 semester hours), Lifetime Fitness (1 semester hour), U.S. Diversity course (3 semester hours), Global Issues course (3 semester hours), English Composition and Rhetoric (6 semester hours).

University of Oklahoma College of Pharmacy

1110 N. Stonewall-Room 133, P.O. Box 26901, Oklahoma City, OK 73190
Phone: (405) 271-6485 **Fax:** (405) 271-3830 **Website:** www.oupharmacy.com
General Info: Public school with an acceptance rate of 33.3% to pharmacy school **Pharmacy Student Body:** 514 **Male/Female Ratio:** 35/65 **Students per Class:** 157 **Joint Degrees Offered:** PharmD/MS in Pharmaceutical Sciences **PCAT:** Required **Minimum Score:** 50% **PharmCAS:** Required **Minimum GPA:** 2.50 **Average GPA:** 3.58 **Application Deadline:** November 1 **Application Fee:** $65 **In-State Tuition:** $9,760 **Out-of-State Tuition:** $13,526 **Prerequisites:** English I and II (6 semester hours), U.S. History (3 semester hours), U.S. Government (3 semester hours), Socio/Behavioral Science (Psychology/Sociology) (3 semester hours), Business Selective (Accounting or Economics) (3 semester hours), Calculus I (3 semester hours), General Physics (3 semester hours), Zoology (4–6 semester hours), Microbiology w/Lab (4 semester hours, pathogenic preferred), General Chemistry I and II (6–8 semester hours), General chemistry I and II w/Lab (2–4 semester hours), Organic Chemistry I and II (6–8 semester hours), Organic Chemistry I and II w/Lab (2–4 semester hours), Human Anatomy or Human Physiology (3 semester hours). General Education requirements: Understanding Art Forms (3 semester hours), Western Civilization and Culture (3 semester hours), Non-Western Civilization and Culture (3 semester hours), Foreign Language I and II (or 2 years of high school language) (6–10 semester hours).

University of Pittsburgh School of Pharmacy

1104 South Salk Hall, 3501 Terrace Street, Pittsburgh, PA 15261
Phone: (412) 624-3270 **Fax:** (412) 648-1086
Website: www.pharmacy.pitt.edu
General Info: Public school with an acceptance rate of 11.6% to pharmacy school. **Pharmacy Student Body:** 395 **Male/Female Ratio:** 39/61 **Students per Class:** 108 **Joint Degrees Offered:** PharmD/MBA, PharmD/JD **PCAT:** Required **Minimum Score:** 50% **PharmCAS:** Required **Minimum GPA:** 3.00 **Average GPA:** 3.65 **Application Deadline:** December 1 **Application Fee:** $65 **In-State Tuition:** $19,620 **Out-of-State Tuition:** $23.630 **Prerequisites:** General Biology I and II w/Lab (8 semester hours), General Chemistry I and II w/Lab (8 semester hours), Organic Chemistry I and II w/Lab (8 semester hours), Calculus (4 semester hours),

Statistics (4 semester hours), Psychology—Introductory (3 semester hours), Economics: intro, macro, micro (3 semester hours), English Composition (6 semester hours), Humanities (6 semester hours), Social Science Electives (6 semester hours), Electives (6 semester hours).

University of Puerto Rico Medical Sciences Campus School of Pharmacy

P.O. Box 365067, San Juan, PR 00936-5067
Phone: (787) 758-2525 ext. 5437
Fax: (787) 751-5860 **Website:** www.upr.clu.edu
General Info: Private school with an acceptance rate of 62.5% to pharmacy school. **Pharmacy Student Body:** 180 **Male/Female Ratio:** 18/82 **Student per Class:** 44 **Joint Degrees Offered:** None **PCAT:** Not specified **PharmCAS:** Not required **Minimum GPA:** N/A **Average GPA:** 3.53 **Application Deadline:** February 9 **Application Fee:** $20 **In-State Tuition:** $3,703 **Out-of-State Tuition:** $7,776 **Prerequisites:** Contact the school and/or visit the website for more information regarding required courses.

University of Rhode Island College of Pharmacy

41 Lower College Road, Kingston, RI 02881
Phone: (401) 874-2761 **Fax:** (401) 874-2181
Website: www.uri.edu/pharmacy/
General Info: Private school with an acceptance rate of 17.5% to pharmacy school **Pharmacy Student Body:** 572 **Male/Female Ratio:** 43/57 **Students per Class:** 94 **Joint Degrees Offered:** PharmD/MS, PharmD/MBA **PCAT:** Not specified **PharmCAS:** Not required **Minimum GPA:** 2.50 **Average GPA:** 3.53 **Application Deadline:** February 1. **Application Fee:** $50 **In-State Tuition:** $5,656 **Out-of-State Tuition:** $19,356 **Prerequisites:** General Chemistry I and II w/Lab (8 credits), Communications (6 credits), General Zoology (4 credits), Organic Chemistry I and II w/Lab (8 credits), Calculus (3 credits), Human Anatomy (4 credits), Microeconomics (3 credits), Intro to Medical Microbiology (4 credits), Intro to Human Physiology w/Lab (4 credits), Biochemistry (3 credits), Intro to Biostatistics (3 credits), Electives (15 credits).

University of the Sciences in Philadelphia College of Pharmacy

600 S. 43rd Street, Philadelphia, PA 19104-4495
Phone: (215) 596-8805 **Fax:** (215) 596-8977

Website: www.usip.edu
General Info: Private school with an acceptance rate of 19.6% to pharmacy school. **Pharmacy Student Body:** 1,579 **Male/Female Ratio:** 35/65 **Students per Class:** 248 **Joint Degrees Offered:** PharmD/MBC, PharmD/JD **PCAT:** Required for applicants seeking admittance into the third-year program **SAT/ACT:** Average scores 1,100/25, respectively (pertains to applicants applying directly out of high school) **PharmCAS:** Not required. **Minimum GPA:** 2.7 **Minimum Science/Math GPA:** 2.3 **Average GPA:** 3.5. **Application Deadline:** January 15. **Application Fee:** $45. **In-State Tuition:** $26,558 **Out-of-State Tuition:** $26,558 **Prerequisites:** General Biology I and II w/Lab, General Chemistry I and II w/Lab, Organic Chemistry I and II w/Lab, Calculus I and II w/Lab, College Composition, Social Science Fundamental Requirement (2 courses), Physics, Microbiology, Speech/Interpersonal Communication, Human Anatomy, Intellectual Heritage I and II. Prerequisites pertinent to students applying to third-year term. High school students do need to have strong science and math background, however. For more information, visit the website above and/or contact the school.

University of Southern California School of Pharmacy

1985 Zonal Avenue, Los Angeles, CA 90089-9121
Phone: (323) 442-1369 **Fax:** (323) 442-1681
Website: www.usd.edu/schools/pharmacy
General Info: Private school with an acceptance rate of 14.7% to pharmacy school. **Pharmacy Student Body:** 745 **Male/Female Ratio:** 25/75 **Students per Class:** 185 **Joint Degrees Offered:** PharmD/MBA, PharmD/MPH, PharmD/JD, PharmD/MS in Regulatory Science, PharmD/MS in Gerontology, PharmD/PhD **PCAT:** Not required **PharmCAS:** Required **Application Deadline:** November 1 **Application Fee:** $85 **In-State Tuition:** $36,172 **Out-of-State Tuition:** $36,172 **Prerequisites:** English (2 semesters), General Chemistry w/Lab (for science majors) (2 semesters), Organic Chemistry w/Lab (for science majors) (2 semesters), General Biology w/Lab (for science majors) (2 semesters), Mammalian Physiology w/Lab (for science majors) (1 semester), Microboiology w/Lab (for science majors) (1 semester), Molecular Biology (for science majors) (1 semester), Biochemistry (for science majors) (1 semester), Physics w/Lab (for science/life science majors) (2 semesters), Calculus (for science majors) (1 semester), Statistics (1 semester), General Psychology or Introductory Sociology (1 semester), Macro- or Microeconomics (1 semester), Interpersonal

Communication (1 semester), Socio/Behavioral Science (nonbaccalaureate holders) (2 semesters), Humanities (nonbaccalaureate holders) (2 semesters).

University of Southern Nevada College of Pharmacy

11 Sunset Way, Henderson, NV 89014
Phone: (702) 968-2017 **Fax:** (702) 990-4435
Website: www.usn.edu
General Info: Private school with an acceptance rate of 10.7% to pharmacy school. **Pharmacy Student Body:** 455 **Male/Female Ratio:** 37/63 **Student/ Faculty Ratio:** 11/1 **Students per Class:** 227 **Full-Time Faculty Members:** 40 **Unique Curriculum Features:** Pharmacy school is a 3-year program, curriculum is divided into a block format rather than semesters/ quarters so that only one class is taken at a time, early pharmacy practice experiences begin in the first week of the program. **Joint Degrees Offered:** PharmD/MBA **PCAT:** Not required **PharmCAS:** Not required **Minimum GPA:** 2.8 **Average GPA:** 3.7 **Early Admissions:** Yes **Application Deadline:** January 12. **Application Fee:** $150 **In-State Tuition:** $36,200 **Out-of-State Tuition:** $36,200 **Prerequisites:** General Chemistry (2 semesters), Organic Chemistry (2 semesters), Microbiology (1 semester), English Composition (1 semester), Speech (1 semester), Calculus (1 semester), Human Anatomy and Physiology (6 semester hours). All applicants must earn a C or better in all prerequisites.

University of Tennessee Health Science Center College of Pharmacy

847 Monroe Avenue, Suite 226, Memphis, TN 38163
Phone: (901) 448-7172 **Fax:** (901) 448-7053
Website: www.uthsc.edu/pharmacy
General Info: Public school with an acceptance rate of 28.6% to pharmacy school. **Pharmacy Student Body:** 551 **Male/Female Ratio:** 42/58 **Students per Class:** 179 **Joint Degrees Offered:** PharmD/PhD **PCAT:** Required **PharmCAS:** Required. **Minimum GPA:** 2.5 **Average GPA:** 3.5 **Application Deadline:** February 1 **Application Fee:** $50 **In-State Tuition:** $11,940 **Out-of-State Tuition:** $24,690 **Prerequisites:** Courses: General Chemistry w/Lab (8 hours), Organic Chemistry w/Lab (8 hours), General Biology/Zoology w/Lab (8 hours), Physics w/Lab (4 hours), Human Anatomy/ Human Physiology w/Lab (8 hours), Microbiology w/Lab (3 hours), Biochemistry w/Lab (6 hours), Immunology (3 hours), Calculus I (3 hours), Statistics (3 hours), English Composition I and II (6 hours),

Communications/Speech (3 hours). Elective Courses: At least 2 courses totaling 6 semester hours in humanities, arts, literature, history, language, philosophy; at least 2 courses totaling 6 semester hours in the social sciences—sociology, psychology, anthropology, political sciences, economics; remaining elective courses totaling 15 hours may be taken in any area(s) the student desires—sciences, mathematics, humanities, or social science. To note: PE, musical performance courses, and ROTC will not be accepted in fulfillment of requirement.

University of Texas–Austin College of Pharmacy

1 University Station A 1900 PHR2.112, Austin, TX 78712-0210
Phone: (512) 471-1737 **Fax:** (512) 471-8783
Website: www.utexas.edu/pharmacy
General Info: A public school with an acceptance rate of 18.1% to pharmacy school. **Pharmacy Student Body:** 520. **Male/Female Ratio:** 26/74 **Students per Class:** 141. **Joint Degrees Offered:** None **PCAT:** Required **PharmCAS:** Not required **Minimum GPA:** 3.00 **Average GPA:** 3.61 **Early Admissions Deadline:** February 1 **Application Deadline:** January 15 **Application Fee:** $75 **In-State Tuition:** $9,918 **Out-of-State Tuition:** $19,168 **Prerequisites:** General Chemistry I and II w/ Lab, Organic Chemistry w/Lab, General Biology I and II w/Lab, Physics I w/Lab, Microbiology w/Lab (General Microbiology: cell structure/genetics and General Microbiology: virology/immunology), Genetics, Calculus, Statistics, English Composition, English Literature.

University of Toledo College of Pharmacy

2801 W. Bancroft Street, Toledo, OH 43606-3390
Phone: (419) 530-1931 **Fax:** (419) 530-1907
Website: www.utpharmacy.org
General Info: Public school with an acceptance rate of 50% to pharmacy school. **Pharmacy Student Body:** 409 **Male/Female Ratio:** 47/53 **Students per Class:** 108 **Joint Degrees Offered:** PharmD/PhD **PCAT:** Not required. GRE Testing: If applicant's GPA is less than 2.7 or applicant is an international student, the GRE test must be taken and submitted. TOEFL Testing: If applicant is an international student from any institution outside the United States, Canada, England, or Australia the TOEFL test will need to be taken and a score of at least 550 is required. **PharmCAS:** Not required. **Minimum GPA:** 3.30 **Average GPA:** 3.37 **Application Deadline:** January 12 **Application Fee:** $40 **In-State Tuition:** $7,899 **Out-of-State Tuition:** $18,180 **Prerequisites:** General Chemistry I and II, General

Biology I and II, Organic Chemistry I and II, Physics I and II, Intro to Pharmacology, Calculus I and II. A minimum of 63 credits must be earned before admittance to the professional division of pharmacy. For further information regarding pharmacy prerequisites, visit the school's website above.

University of Utah College of Pharmacy

30 S. 2000 East, Room 201, Salt Lake City, UT 84112-5820
Phone: (801) 581-6731 **Fax:** (801) 51-3716
Website: www.pharmacy.utah.edu
General Info: Public school with an acceptance rate of 28.6% to pharmacy school. **Pharmacy Student Body:** 182 **Male/Female Ratio:** 39/61 **Students per Class:** 51 **Joint Degrees Offered:** PharmD/PhD **PCAT:** Required **Minimum Score:** 65% **PharmCAS:** Not required **Minimum GPA:** 2.75 **Average GPA:** 3.50 **Application Deadline:** January 10 **Application Fee:** $105 **In-State Tuition:** $10,604 **Out-of-State Tuition:** $22,690 **Prerequisites:** General Chemistry w/Lab (1 year), Organic Chemistry w/Lab (1 year), Calculus (1 year) Physics (1 year), Human Anatomy (1 semester),Human Physiology (1 semester),Professional/Technical Writing (1 semester), Microbiology (1 semester).

University of Washington School of Pharmacy

H364 Health Sciences, Box 357631, Seattle, WA 98195-7631
Phone: (206) 543-2030 **Fax:** (206) 685-9297
Website: http://depts.wasington.edu/pha
General Info: Public school with an acceptance rate of 20% to pharmacy school. **Pharmacy Student Body:** 350 **Male/Female Ratio:** 29/71 **Students per Class:** 86. **Joint Degrees Offered:** PharmD/PhD, PharmD/MS in Pharmaceutical Outcomes and Policy, PharmD/PA **PCAT:** Required **Minimum Score:** 60% in Chemistry; 25% in other areas **PharmCAS:** Required **Minimum GPA:** 3.0 **Average GPA:** 3.6 **Application Deadline:** January 5. **Application Fee:** $45 **In-State Tuition:** $14,754 **Out-of-State Tuition:** $28,663 **Prerequisites:** English Composition (6–8 semester hours), General Chemistry (8 semester hours), Organic Chemistry (8 semester hours), General Biology (8 semester hours), Microbiology (4 semester hours), Calculus (4 semester hours), Statistics (4 semester hours), Humanities Electives (7–8 semester hours), Social Science Electives (7—8 semester hours).

University of Wisconsin–Madison School of Pharmacy

777 Highland Avenue, Madison, WI 53705-2222
Phone: (608) 262-1414 **Fax:** (608) 262-3397
Website: www.pharmacy.wisc.edu/
General Info: Public school with an acceptance rate of 33% to pharmacy school. **Pharmacy Student Body:** 520 **Male/Female Ratio:** 45/55 **Students per Class:** 161 **Student/Faculty Ratio:** 9/1 **Joint Degrees Offered:** PharmD/JD, PharmD/MBA, PharmD/MPH, PharmD/PhD or MS **PCAT:** Required with a composite score of 86 **PharmCAS:** Not required **Minimum GPA:** N/A **Average GPA:** 3.6 **Application Deadline:** December 1 **Application Fee:** $45 **In-State Tuition:** $13,124 year 4: $16,500 **Out-of-State Tuition:** $25,582 **Prerequisites:** Biology w/Lab (8 credits), Chemistry w/Lab (8 credits), Organic Chemistry w/Lab (8 credits), College Physics w/Lab (8 credits), Calculus (for science majors) (4–5 credits), Communication, Microeconomics (3 credits), Social Science (3 credits), Behavioral Science (3 credits), Ethnic Studies (3 credits). Other college courses to bring total to 62 credits.

University of Wyoming School of Pharmacy

1000 E. University Avenue, Department 3375, Laramie, WY 82071
Phone: (307) 766-6132 **Fax:** (307) 766-2953
Website: www.uwyo.edu/pharmacy
General Info: Public school with an acceptance rate of 8.3% to pharmacy school. **Pharmacy Student Body:** 208 **Male/Female Ratio:** 26/74 **Students per Class:** 52 **Student/Faculty Ratio:** 14/1 **Joint Degrees Offered:** None **PCAT:** Required **Minimum Score:** 50% **PharmCAS:** Required **Minimum GPA:** 2.8 **Average GPA:** 3.6 **Application Deadline:** February 1 **Application Fee:** $50 **In-State Tuition:** $25,635 **Out-of-State Tuition:** $38,555 **Prerequisites:** Human Anatomy and Physiology (8 semester hours), General Biology w/Lab (8 semester hours), General Chemistry w/Lab (8 semester hours), Microbiology w/Lab (4 semester hours), Organic Chemistry w/Lab (8 semester hours), Physics w/Lab (4 semester hours), Statistics (2 semester hours), Precalculus Algebra (3 semester hours), Calculus (3 semester hours), Ethics (3 semester hours, Economics (3 semester hours), English Composition (6 semester hours), Psychology or Sociology (3 semester hours), History or Political Science (3 semester hours).

Virginia Commonwealth University at the Medical College of Virginia Campus School of Pharmacy

410 N. 12th Street, Room 155, Smith Building, Richmond, VA 23298-0581
Phone: (804) 828-3006 **Fax:** (804) 827-0002
Website: www.pharmacy.vcu.edu
General Info: Public School with an acceptance rate of 10.4% to pharmacy school. **Pharmacy Student Body:** 449 **Male/Female Ratio:** 30/70 **Students per Class:** 129 **Joint Degrees Offered:** PharmD/MS, PharmD/MBA, PharmD/MPH, PharmD/PhD **PCAT:** Required **PharmCAS:** Required **Minimum GPA:** N/A **Average GPA:** 3.5 **Early Admissions Deadline:** September 1 **Application Deadline:** March 1 **Application Fee:** N/A **In-State Tuition:** $11,211 **Out-of-State Tuition:** $15,316 **Prerequisites:** English (6 semester hours), General Chemistry (lecture and lab) (8 semester hours), Organic Chemistry (lecture and lab) (8 semester hours), General Biology (lecture and lab) (8 semester hours), Physics (lecture and lab) (8 semester hours), Mathematics (9 semester hours), Public Speaking (3 semester hours), Electives (18 semester hours).

Washington State University College of Pharmacy

P.O. Box 646510, Pullman, WA 99164-6510
Phone: (509) 335-4750 **Fax:** (509) 335-2530
Website: www.pharmacy.wsu.edu
General Info: Public School with an acceptance rate of 10% to pharmacy school. **Pharmacy Student Body:** 358 **Male/Female Ratio:** 33/67 **Students per Class:** 95 **Joint Degrees Offered:** None **PCAT:** Not required **PharmCAS:** Required. **Average GPA:** 3.6 **Application Deadline:** January 5 **Application Fee:** $50 **In-State Tuition:** $15,450 **Out-of-State Tuition:** $29,284 **Prerequisites:** Principles of Chemistry I and II (8 semester hours), Organic Chemistry I and II w/Lab (7 semester hours), Introductory to Biology I and II (8 semester hours), Calculus (4 semester hours), Microbiology (3 semester hours), Biochemistry (upper division) (4 semester hours), World Civilization (6 semester hours), Social Sciences/Arts and Humanities (9 semester hours), Written and Speech Communications (6 semester hours), Cultural Studies (3 semester hours), Tier III Capstone (a graduation requirement, must be a 400-level and may be completed during the first professional year at WSU) (3 semester hours).

Wayne State University Eugene Applebaum College of Pharmacy Health and Sciences

259 Mack Avenue, Suite 1600, Detroit, MI 48201
Phone: (313) 577-1716 **Fax:** (313) 577-0457
Website: www.cphs.wayne.edu
General Info: Public school with an acceptance rate of 1.3% to pharmacy school. **Pharmacy Student Body:** 279 **Male/Female Ratio:** 33/67 **Students per Class:** 88 **Joint Degrees Offered:** PharmD/PhD **PCAT:** Required. **PharmCAS:** Required **Minimum GPA:** 2.80 **Average GPA:** 3.62 **Application Deadline:** December 1 **Application Fee:** $50 **In-State Tuition:** $17,017 **Out-of-State Tuition:** $28,529 **Prerequisites:** Biology (general/basic life mechanisms), Introduction to Microbiology, Chemical Structure and Bonds, General/Organic Chemistry, Organic Chemistry, Calculus I, General Physics I, Computer Literacy, English Proficiency, Critical Thinking Competency, Economics, Introduction to College Writing, Intermediate Writing, Introduction to American Government, Basic Speech.

Western University of Health Sciences College of Pharmacy

309 E. 2nd Street, Pomona, CA 91766-1854
Phone: (909) 469-5581 **Fax:** (909) 469-5539
Website: www.westernu.edu
General Info: Private school with an acceptance rate of 10.3% to pharmacy school. **Pharmacy Student Body:** 438 **Male/Female Ratio:** 20/80 **Students per Class:** 120 **Joint Degrees Offered:** PharmD/MS **PCAT:** Not required. **PharmCAS:** Required **Minimum GPA:** 2.5 **Average GPA:** 3.39 **Application Deadline:** November 1 **Application Fee:** $65 **In-State Tuition:** $34,030 **Out-of-State Tuition:** $34,030 **Prerequisites:** English (3 semester hours), English Composition (3 semester hours), General Chemistry w/Lab (8 semester hours), Organic Chemistry w/Lab (8 semester hours), Human Anatomy w/Lab (4 semester hours), Human Physiology w/Lab, Microbiology w/Lab (4 semester hours), Biochemistry (lab optional) (6 semester hours), Speech Communication (3 semester hours), Calculus (3 semester hours), Elective 1 (3 semester hours), Elective 2 (3 semester hours).

West Virginia University School of Pharmacy

P.O. Box 9500, 1136 Health Sciences North, Morgantown, WV 26506-9500
Phone: (304) 293-5101 **Fax:** (304) 293-5483
Website: www.hsc.wvu.edu/sop

General Info: Public school with an acceptance rate of 17.5% to pharmacy school. **Pharmacy Student Body:** 316 **Male/Female Ratio:** 40/60 **Students per Class:** 80 **Joint Degrees Offered:** PharmD/MS, PharmD/PhD **PCAT:** Required **PharmCAS:** Required. **Application Deadline:** December 1 **Application Fee:** $50 **In-State Tuition:** $15,792 **Out-of-State Tuition:** $26,890 **Prerequisites:** English Composition (6 semester hours), General Chemistry (8 semester hours), Organic Chemistry (8 semester hours), General Biology (8 semester hours), General Microbiology (3 semester hours), Introduction to Calculus (3 semester hours), Physics (8 semester hours), Principles of Microeconomics (3 semester hours), Introduction to Statistics (3 semester hours), Humanities and Fine Arts (12 semester hours), Social and Behavioral Sciences (6 semester hours).

Wingate University School of Pharmacy

316 N. Main Street, Campus Box 3087, Wingate, NC 28174
Phone: (702) 233-8331 **Fax:** (704) 233-8332
Website: www.wingate.edu
General Info: Private school with an acceptance rate of 7.8% to pharmacy school. **Pharmacy Student Body:** 179. **Male/Female Ratio:** 40/60 **Students per Class:** 70 **Joint Degrees Offered:** PharmD/MBA **PCAT:** Required **Minimum Score:** 50% **PharmCAS:** Required **Minimum GPA:** 3.0 **Average GPA:** 3.7 **Application Deadline:** February 2 **Application Fee:** $25 **In-State Tuition:** $21,890 **Out-of-State Tuition:** $25,260 **Prerequisites:** English Composition/Literature (6 semester hours), General Chemistry w/Lab (8 semester hours), Organic Chemistry w/Lab (8 semester hours), Biology w/Lab (8 semester hours), General Microbiology w/Lab (4 semester hours), Physics (4 semester hours), Calculus (3 semester hours), Statistics (3 semester hours), Speech (public speaking) (3 semester hours), Economics (3 semester hours), Humanities/Social Sciences (9 semester hours), Other (3 semester hours). One course in anatomy is recommended but not required. Psychology, Sociology, Foreign Language, and Philosophy are not required but are highly recommended to satisfy the Humanities/Social Sciences requirement.

Xaiver University of Louisiana College of Pharmacy

#1 Drexel Drive, New Orleans, LA 70125
Phone: (504) 520-7421 **Fax:** (504) 520-7930
Website: www.xula.edu/pharmacy
General Info: Private school with an acceptance rate of 12.5% to pharmacy school. **Pharmacy Student Body:** 590 **Male/Female Ratio:** 29/71 **Students per Class:** 165 **Joint Degrees Offered:** None **PCAT:** Required **PharmCAS:** Not required **Minimum GPA:** 2.5 **Average GPA:** 3.2 **Application Deadline:** December 15 **Application Fee:** $20 **In-State Tuition:** $19,600 **Out-of-State Tuition:** $19,600 **Prerequisites:** Biology (11 semester credits), Chemistry (16 semester credits), Physics (3 semester credits), Psychology or Sociology (3 semester credits), Economics (3 semester credits), Speech Communication (3 semester credits), English (6 semester credits), Theology (3 semester credits), Mathematics (8 semester credits), Academic Elective (3 semester credits), Philosophy (6 semester credits).

Works Cited

Hodges KA. "Web-based Program Broadens Medicare Part D Services: Pharmacists Provide MTM Services to Community Care Rx Patients." *Pharmacy Today*, 12/2006, 29-31.

Morse R and Flanigan S. "Best Graduate Schools: Health Rankings Methodology." http://www.usnews.com/articles/education/best-graduate-schools/2009/04/22/health-rankings-methodology.html, April 15, 2010.

Bureau of Labor Statistics, U.S. Department of Labor, *Occupational Outlook Handbook, 2010–2011 Edition*, Pharmacists. http://www.bls.gov/oco/ocos079.htm (accessed October 2010).

Bureau of Labor Statistics, Occupational Employment Statistics for May 2009. http://www.bls.gov/oes/current/oes291051.htm (accessed October 2010)

The Adequacy of Pharmacist Supply: 2004 to 2030. Department of Health and Human Services, Health Resources and Services Administration (HRSA), Bureau of Health Professions, December 2008. http://bhpr.hrsa.gov/healthworkforce/pharmacy/ (accessed October 2010)

In addition to pharmacy school websites, the following websites were consulted:

www.aacp.org

www.accp.com

www.acpe-accredit.org

www.aphanet.org

www.ashp.org

www.bpsweb.org

www.pharmacymanpower.com

www.nabp.net

www.nacds.org

www.ncpanet.org

www.pcatweb.info

www.pharmcas.org

www.pharmacist.com

INDEX